6-18-69

JOHNNY

By the Same Author

Jeanie O'Brien

JOHNNY

Owenita Sanderlin

South Brunswick and New York:
A. S. Barnes and Company
London: Thomas Yoseloff Ltd

A. S. Barnes and Co., Inc.

Cranbury, New Jersey 08512

Thomas Yoseloff Ltd

18 Charing Cross Road

London, W.C. 2, England

The author is grateful to the Houghton Mifflin
Company, for permission to reprint material from
The Hobbit, by J. R. R. Tolkien, which appears
in Chapter 2

6766

Printed in the United States of America

1496721

Contents

JOHNNY

1

A Walk on the Beach

I WENT IN AND SAT DOWN ON THE STOOL NEXT TO THE DESK
with the nurse looking into a microscope, counting cells.
I did that at the hospital clinic every other Saturday, unless my mom could argue Dr. Evans into letting me off
for a tournament.

It wasn't that they wouldn't let me play tennis. I've
had this trouble with my blood ever since about three
years ago, when I was eleven years old, but all I had to
do was take pills and I was okay. They said I could do
anything as long as my red count stayed up, but they
had to keep checking. And Dr. Evans was an internationally known hematologist so you could hardly expect him
to arrange his hours to suit an internationally unknown
boy. But my mom did.

"How's the tennis?" Thelma said, and I said "Great.
We're going to the Nationals!"

Thelma was the lab technician who had gotten polio
when she was my age and has to wear braces. That was
before Dr. Salk developed the polio vaccine so hardly
anybody gets polio anymore. I think doctors are great

but I wouldn't want to be one. Imagine having to spend all that time in a hospital.

I kept telling Thelma about the guys I knew at the public parks who played good tennis with braces, or with just one arm or leg, and she ought to try it. But she said she'd better stick to her knitting. Not that I ever saw her doing any knitting. We kidded each other a lot.

When I first started going to the clinic three years ago, I wasn't even as big as Thelma, who is about as big as a bird. Now I was lots taller than she was, and my weight was up from 89 to 120. I did pushups every day and I was really getting strong. Every time I went there I hoped maybe this time Dr. Evans would say I didn't have to come back again.

I didn't mind getting my finger stuck; it was the waiting around afterwards that was so boring. Mom and I would sit in the waiting room at the end of the corridor where you could look out a big window at the ocean. I sure like the ocean. It's the most beautiful thing in the world, I guess, although of course I haven't seen much of the world yet. My father is writing a book about the first ship that sailed around the globe and that's the way I'd like to travel, by sea. You won't catch me going on an airplane. I found that out when I had to fly to a medical convention so all the doctors could look at the Boy Wonder who has whatever I have wrong with me. My mom says they can't figure it out, and maybe some day I'll be famous. Big deal. I'd rather play tennis.

Waiting was harder than ever that day because Dad and David, my brother, were sitting in the car in front of the hospital with all our stuff packed to take off for Kalamazoo the minute Mom got Dr. Evans to say it would be okay for me to go. Kalamazoo, Michigan, is where they have the National Junior and Boys tennis championships every year in July, and this year David had a good chance to win. My parents still wouldn't let me play singles in big tournaments, but I could play doubles, and my friend Roy and I had won all the Southern California tournaments in our age division, fourteen and under, so we had a chance, too.

Dr. Evans usually came down the hall at about twelve o'clock and boomed out, "Well, Johnny? Off to the Tennis Wars?" But that day he didn't come. He sent his new assistant, Dr. Granville, who wasn't very old and didn't know the ropes yet. Thelma said I wore out more new assistants than any other patient they ever had; she said probably I'd be the next one myself, but I said *no thanks*.

"Dr. Evans said it would be all right for you to leave now, John," this doctor said. "And he would like to see you for a moment in his office," he said to my mom.

"What's my count?" I demanded.

The new ones always refuse to tell me my blood count. What the heck do they think I've been sitting there for all morning? I keep a chart of it, and I like to know.

"We are not at liberty to divulge that information," Dr. Granville said, or something stuffy like that. Like calling me "John." *Nobody* calls me John.

"You go on out and tell Dad I'll be right out," Mom said. She had that glint in her eye that she gets when she's about to go in and do battle. Sometimes Dr. Evans wants me to come back in one week, and that would wreck everything. She was planning on trying for three, so we could stop by the Grand Canyon on our way back home.

Maybe I'd get even longer; anyhow, I always shot out of that old clinic as fast as I could walk, and I can walk pretty fast, so I did. It's so good to get through that stale sick smell; out front, I breathed my lungs full of good fresh air that tasted like ice cold pop, after three sets of singles.

"Hey, Johnny!" David yelled at me from across the street. "We had to move the car."

"Where's Mom?" Dad said. Poor Dad. He doesn't know it, but when he gets worried, he gets this desperate glare on his face. I sure hope I never worry as much as he does.

"Relax," I said, and burrowed in with the baggage on the back seat. "She's just talking Dr. Evans into an extra week."

Dad and David had been practicing at some tennis courts which are conveniently located across from the clinic; and they were still pretty sweaty. They look a lot alike, tall—Dad's over six feet and Dave is getting there— and they both get this nice dark tan all over which never burns the way I do. I have sandy colored hair like my sisters', and I get pink.

I have two sisters, Frea and Mary, but they are married and having babies now. Whenever you start talking about tennis, they get this polite glaze over their eyes which everybody does who isn't interested in it. But Dad and Mom and David and I spend all our spare time on the courts, or else we're swinging our rackets around in the living room showing each other how we do our strokes, except Mom, who just gets the ball back any old way she can. Mom says David and I climbed out of our play pens onto the tennis court, and were talking about forehands and backhands before we could tell right hands from left hands. We sure have a lot of fun.

"I think I'll go see if Mom's coming," Dad said.

I knew it wouldn't do any good to try to stop him, but he hates hospitals worse than I do so I said, "It's a lot nicer out here."

But he went.

David said, "I heard Roy won the boys' singles at Kentucky State, so probably you two will be seeded in the doubles at the Nationals."

Roy is my best friend and doubles partner. We have been playing together ever since we were ten years old.

"Seeded" means you are supposed to be one of the best teams and you won't have to play the other top teams until the semi-finals and finals. It sure would be neat if we were!

But now I was wondering—my mother was staying in there so long. And I began to wish Dad hadn't gone in, because he was apt to say something like "What if it's hot back East? I don't think Johnny ought to play in that heat."

The only time I ever heard my parents having a fight was after my blood count got back up to normal after the first time I was sick, and the doctor said I could play all the tennis I wanted to and Dad said I had to wait a year and Mom said that was ridiculous and it finally ended up with the Great Compromise; I could play easy singles, for practice, and doubles in tournaments.

As long as my count was okay.

Mom and Dad were coming out of the front door of the hospital, and Mom was trying to look cheerful. It isn't as easy to tell what my mother is thinking as it is to tell about Dad, and she used to be able to fool me— but not after three years of taking me to the clinic every two weeks, with side trips to Berkeley to see the doctors at The University of California.

So I knew, even before they got across the street, that I wasn't going to be able to go to the Nationals.

They had to wait for a break in the traffic. My throat was so swelled up I couldn't talk, and it was a good thing I couldn't because I was full of mean thoughts. I didn't want David to go, if I couldn't. I was only getting to play doubles anyway, and he could play singles all the time. Why did I have to be sick, and David well? And Roy, back there winning the boys' singles in Kentucky. Before I got sick I could beat Roy easy—why did God let me get sick? I even blamed God, I was so mad.

I got out of the car on the sidewalk side, and walked away. I heard Mom calling "Johnny!" but I didn't listen.

Then she didn't call anymore, and I kept on walking. I crossed the street and went down the hill to the beach. The sand was glaring white and the ocean blurred...

I was way down the beach, on the wet sand, when there was my dad, walking along beside me. He didn't say anything; we just walked, stepping over piles of seaweed, watching the sea gulls flap away when we got too close, and listening to the surf. We went all the way to the oceanography pier and back, and it felt good, walking along with my dad.

Mom was sitting in the car with David. I could tell she had been crying but she was trying to look as if she hadn't. She has brown eyes and short, curly brown hair and is very young-looking for a grandmother. I sure have a nice family.

"Listen, David," I said. "You have to go. Even if I can't, you have to."

David and I live in the same room, but we still get along great. That's because when I was born he was so

glad I was a boy. Frea and Mary are nice, but who wants
to be a boy with three sisters?

"You have to," I said.

"Okay," David said.

"And *win*."

"Yep," he said.

"Okay."

2

"A Number of Things"

"The World is so full of a number of things,
I'm sure we should all be as happy as kings."

I BET ROBERT LOUIS STEVENSON WAS SICK WHEN HE WROTE
that. He was sick a lot of the time, and that's when you
find out how much there is to do that you never thought
of before.

When I'm okay, there's only one thing in the world I
want to do: play tennis.

But if I can't play tennis, I just have to think of something else. So I thought of a lot of things to do that summer, while David was gone to the Nationals. I couldn't
wait to get up every morning, there was so much I wanted
to do.

The first thing after I got home from the hospital—
where I had to have a couple of transfusions—my parents
told me I could have anything I wanted, to make up for
not getting to go back East.

"Just so we can afford it," Mom said.

I said I'd like to think it over for a while, and they

said sure, take as long as I wanted, and my Dad said he was teaching the summer session in August so we *could* afford it, whatever it was.

The morning after Dr. Evans let me go home, I woke up early and lay there in bed a long time, looking around the room. It was a wide bed, big enough for me and David, but it was kind of nice being able to roll over all I wanted to, which you certainly can't do in a hospital bed or even if you're sleeping with your brother.

And all of a sudden I realized I wouldn't be sleeping with David anymore, because he was going away to college in the fall. At first I felt sad, but then I got kind of interested.

If it was my bed, and my room, I could do anything I wanted to with it. I could fix it up.

Having two boys in one room can get rather messy, so the first thing I did after breakfast was to clean it out. There were about a million old tennis balls in the closet so I put them in bags. I found out in *World Tennis* magazine where you can sell old tennis balls so I decided to make some money while I was about it. I have various other money-making schemes, like saving up pennies, which practically everybody will give you if you are saving them; and lending money to anyone in the family for one cent per one dollar every ten days; and even baby-sitting, but only for my sisters' babies.

Mom was poking her head in from time to time, to see if I needed any help cleaning my room, so I let her do the dusting. We put David's school papers, which were all over the place, in a cardboard carton—"I expect he'll just throw them away," Mom said, "but we'll let him decide"—and then we sorted out our outgrown clothes to send to the Little Indian tribe in South Dakota, and I found a couple of neat shirts of David's that would fit me now, and a practically new pair of pajamas.

"Do you know what they call those horrible white things they make you wear in the hospital? I asked my mom. "*Johnnies*!"

That's the most disgusting thing I have ever heard of.

After lunch I sorted out all our collections. David said before he left that I could have his stamps and coins, because he wouldn't have time for stuff like that anymore, and I had almost two thousand post cards. I decided to arrange them by states and countries, and keep a record of how many I had for each one. I put them in a shoe box, which is a neat place for a postcard collection as they just fit.

We have a bunch of books about tennis in our bookcase and I decided to read them. They looked pretty interesting but ordinarily I don't have much time to read. We had some good ones on chess too. After supper my Dad and I played chess. We have a big polished wood set that my parents brought from Mexico for Christmas. The pieces are about six inches to a foot high, and hand-carved.

"If I can have anything in the world I want," I told Dad during one of those long pauses while he is thinking what to do next and I have already decided on my next three moves, "I'd pick this chess set, only we already have it."

Dad grinned at me and moved his horse. It wasn't what I'd figured him to do so I had to change my plans. Still, after a long hard struggle, I managed to beat him.

Dad and Mom and David and I all play chess in different ways. Dad is like the turtle in the Hare and the Tortoise. Mom admits that she never thinks more than one move ahead and the only time she ever won was by accident; she had me checkmated and I had to tell her! Not that Mom is stupid; she just doesn't have that kind of a brain. I like math and that's the way I play chess, like solving problems. But David is the champ; you ought to see him play chess. He tears right out after your king, and never mind what happens to his men on the way. That's the way he plays tennis too. And pingpong. I'm pretty good at pingpong, but I can't beat him. When he comes home, I'll be the champion of nothing.

My room looked great when I went to bed that night, but after I turned off the light and rolled over a couple of times, just to see how good it felt having it all to myself, I got this big lump in my throat and I wished David would hurry up and come home. Even if our room was messy, and I'd have to be runner-up all the time.

Then I thought how it used to be when Frea and Mary were in the next room, giggling and shrieking with a bunch of their girl friends; or when Frea and Mary and David and I used to sleep out on the porch, and Frea told us scary stories. Now they were married, and would never come back, and it would be the same way with David. He would go to college, and meet some girl . . .

The house was so quiet, I could hear the faucet dripping, out in the kitchen, but then I listened harder and I could hear my dad's old typewriter tap-tapping away, a mile a minute, at the other end of the house, and I felt better.

The next day I decided to start a newspaper, and established my office in my room. It would come out every week, and cover all my activities. After considerable thought I named it "The Spy."

Banner headline in the first issue was DAVID GOES

TO NATIONALS. Others were "Paper Office Established," "Doctors Foiled by White Count," "Weight-lifting Record Set," "The Absent Minded Professor" (a neat movie we saw), and "Hot Spell" (the weather). I also had a few ads—"Need Money? Try Tellson's" and "Expert Name-Carving" (on racket handles). When I asked Dad what to write about for an editorial, he said the best thing is to think of your pet gripes, and that was easy. Hospital beds!

"Hospital beds should be improved! Hospital beds are more uncomfortable than any I have ever slept on. They are too high for one thing, and also too narrow. If you turn over you may find yourself on the floor. They are also too hard. My bed at home is relatively firm, but feels soft compared to the hospital bed, which curves upward into your spine. I would rather sleep on top of Snoopy's doghouse."

Then I got one of my Peanuts books and traced a picture of Snoopy lying on his back on the doghouse roof saying. "Who wouldn't?"

He looked pretty cute. Boy, if I could draw like Schulz I'd really have it made.

The next Saturday, Dad didn't have to teach summer school, so we had a picnic at the beach. We took Frea's two little girls, Kathy and Teri, and Mary's little boys, Bryan and Craig, and I showed them how to build sandcastles, and tied strings of seaweed around their waists, and covered them up with sand, and chased waves down at the edge of the water. It's fun to do things like that with little kids; they get so excited, and laugh and shriek, and fall down and look funny. I still can't get over hearing them call me *Uncle* Johnny.

Then Dad and Mom took turns babysitting so we could go out and jump over the waves. Mom and I went first; I get a kick out of Mom because the minute she gets into the ocean you wouldn't think she is a grown-up.

"Here comes a big one!" she screams. "Come on! Let's get out there."

So we churn our way out as fast as we can go, trying to make it before the wave breaks, and then "Whee!" Mom yells, and we go up and over and it sure is fun.

"Watch out!" I yell back. "Here comes another one. This is a monster."

Then it's Dad's turn, and I go back and find him stretched out on a towel on the sand.

"Come on, Dad!" I say, pulling him up.

"Haven't you had enough yet?" he protests.

"What's the matter?" I tease. "You getting too old, Dad?"

So he grumbles some more, but he always goes, and when we get out there he says, "Gee, this is great!" and we jump over about seven waves, with every one getting bigger than the last, and we are both having the best time we ever had in our lives when he gets that worried look on his face and says "We better go in."

"Aw, Dad—just one more?" I beg, but I am shivering and I know he's right, so we go in.

After you get home from the beach, you feel so good —nice and clean, without having to take a bath, and cool and sleepy. After supper, which was fried chicken, and boy, was I hungry, we went out to Dad's study and read *The Hobbit*, by J. R. Tolkien; this was our third time through. It's a very good book for reading out loud, for instance where the dwarves were washing the hobbit's dishes for him, and he squeaked with fright "Please be careful! Please don't trouble! I can manage," and they sang,

> Chip the glasses and crack the plates,
> Blunt the knives and bend the forks,
> That's what Bilbo Baggins hates,
> Smash the bottles, and burn the corks.

I wrote a book report on it for school back in junior high; usually I hate book reports because you are supposed to read something "worthwhile" and then pretend that it is fascinating and everybody ought to read it, when you really think it is boring. But *The Hobbit* is my favorite book so here is what it's all about in case you want to read it:

THE HOBBIT

The Hobbit is a book filled with suspense and comedy. It starts when a wizard, Gandalf, visits the hobbit and convinces him into being a burglar for some elves who want to regain their gold which Smaug, a dragon, has stolen from them and is now guarding. In case you are wondering just what a hobbit is I will tell you. A hobbit is like a man, except smaller. This particular hobbit is a very round, honest-looking one and he never gets surprised—until he goes on this adventure.

That was the first time I ever got an A on a book report so I think it ought to be framed! I guess the secret of it is you have to really like the book, and I never liked to read much until this summer, when I couldn't play tennis.

David sent me another book that I liked very much. It was about the famous tennis player, Billy Talbert, who became a national champion even though he had diabetes and had to take insulin. He said playing tennis helped him, and other people who had diabetes should not be afraid to try it. The name of this book was *Playing For Life*.

Two weeks after I got out of the hospital my blood count was back up to normal. Unfortunately, the new pills I had to take were terrible. They made my face swell up so I looked like a fat boy with the mumps. Dr. Evans said this was only temporary, but I sure didn't like it. However, the important thing was, I could play tennis again.

I shot out of the clinic and broke the news to my dad. It was a great day anyway, because David was in the semi-finals at Kalamazoo and we could hardly wait for him to call up long distance at six o'clock and tell us if he won. I was sure he was going to win.

"How about stopping by the tennis courts?" I told Dad. "Dr. Evans says I'm okay."

"Great," Dad said. "But I have a couple of tickets to the ball game this afternoon."

"The Padres!" I said. "Oh boy. I guess I can wait one more day to play tennis."

The ball game between the San Diego Padres and Seattle was really close. It was another beautiful day, with the sun shining and a breeze rippling the flag, and the Padres came through with the tying run in the bottom of the ninth, so we got to see an extra inning and then the Padres won. It was perfect.

And when we got home, the phone was ringing and they let me answer.

"It's David! It's David!" I cried. My heart was beating so loud I could hardly hear him. "He won! He won! Here, Mom, you can talk to him. Hurry up, Dad! ask him who's in the finals!"

I was so happy that night I couldn't go to sleep. I lay awake in my wide bed in the dark room, with moonlight shining in the window and the night birds singing, and said my prayers. Usually I get lost in the middle, but this night I said Amen, and I was still awake.

After a while Mom came in and I said, "Hi, Mom!"

"You awake?" she whispered.

"I'm so happy I can't go to sleep," I said. "You know what?"

She sat down on my bed and smoothed my hair back. "What, honey?"

"I think this must be what it's like in heaven. I mean, the way I feel."

"I guess it is," Mom said. "And you're such a good boy, you're bound to go there some day."

"Gee, thanks, Mom," I said. "You better watch out. My head's swelled up enough already!" I didn't mind about my face anymore. I could even make a joke about it. I was lucky they had some pills that would let me play tennis again.

"And you know what else?" I said. "There isn't anything in the world that I want, so you won't have to spend any money."

Mom leaned over and kissed me on the forehead.

"I love you," she said, and I said, "Likewise."

3

Black Sunday

UP TO THE TIME I WAS EIGHT YEARS OLD WE LIVED IN THE
state of Maine, which they say is "Nine months winter
and three months poor sleddin'."

We all had a good time there, picking apples and visiting the cows at the university barns, and building snow
forts and cutting down our own Christmas tree in the
pine grove. I played my first tennis tournament at North-
east Harbor when I was seven; David taught me how to
serve in one week so I could be in it. I didn't win because the lowest age division they had was thirteen and
under, but David won it when he was ten.

After that we moved to California and boy, was it
different! Eleven months summer and one month poor
swimmin'.

The house we picked, out in the back country near
El Cajon, was really neat. It's what they call early California ranch style, all on one floor with a gallery outside,
with brick floors and wooden posts that have flowers
with ridiculous names like begonias and bougainvilleas

growing up them, and this gallery surrounds a back yard which out West is called a patio, with a pepper tree in the middle of it. A pepper tree looks like a weeping willow, only it has little red berries on it besides the drippy green leaves.

Our hill, which is surrounded by uninhabited mountains, has a lot of pepper trees on it, and also many other kinds of trees which you would never find back East, such as olive, tangerine, palm, orange, grapefruit, lemon and lime trees; and the dirt road which winds up the hill to our house is lined with eucalyptus, which are about the tallest, skinniest trees there are. We also have a large variety of interesting cactus plants, which my dad won't go within ten feet of because he claims they reach out and stick him.

The inside of our house starts with a living room at one end, and from there you have to walk through a kitchen, a hall with two bedrooms and a bath off of it, through another bedroom to get to my dad's study, at the other end. This works out very well for watching TV, which we couldn't have in Maine, when Dad's room was on top of the living room and Mom had to keep telling us "Sssh! *Daddy's working!*"

The way our house happened to stretch out this way was by accident; it started many years ago with just the middle, and then different people who owned it added on at both ends. But I recommend this floor plan for a family with several children and a father who likes to study. I like to draw plans for houses. I might decide to be an architect, if I don't teach math or be a tennis pro.

That Sunday morning when David was playing in the finals of the Nationals, I got up early because when it was eight o'clock in San Diego it would be ten o'clock in Kal-

amazoo, and he might be starting to play his singles.
Of course, he might not play them until later—maybe
one o'clock? I wished we had asked him when.

"Come on, David!" I went around muttering to myself.
"Come on!" And when we went to church, I said prayers
for him, although I don't usually pray for stuff like winning games when the world is in such bad shape.

Dad and Mom felt just like I did. Mom said she was
too excited to cook dinner so we went to the Chuck
Wagon, where you can eat all you want to and usually I
stuff myself, but we couldn't eat much either, that day.

Then we hurried home to be near the phone when
David called—but he didn't call.

It got later and later. In July, it stays light until eight
o'clock, which would be ten o'clock back there.

"I don't understand it," Mom said. "He wasn't in the
doubles finals, so he *must* be through."

"Maybe it rained," I said.

"Maybe he lost," Dad said, in a voice like Eeyore.

"It *must* have rained—why don't you call the newspaper?" Mom suggested.

Dad was just looking up the number when the phone
rang.

Mom let me answer, but it wasn't David. It was Roy.

"Hi, Johnny," he said.

"Roy! Where are you?"

"I just got home. We flew back."

It was great hearing Roy's voice; I'd missed him almost as much as David.

"How did you do?" I asked.

"We lost," he said. "You should have been there, Johnny. It would have been a cinch."

I thought I'd got over feeling bad about it, but I couldn't

even talk; my throat was stuck. It wasn't not being the national champion I minded as much as missing all the fun of it, with Roy. We always had such a great time together.

"We'll win it next year," he said.

"Sure."

"What about David?" Mom whispered. "Does he know anything about David?"

"Roy? What about David?"

"Just a minute," he said.

Then he didn't say anything for a while and then Bob said, "Hi, Johnny!" Bob is Roy's father, and next to my dad he's the greatest.

"How did David do?" I asked. I was beginning to feel scared, and I knew there was something wrong when he said, "Let me speak to your father."

Dad listened for a long time, and then he said, "Thanks for calling, Bob. You're sure he's all right?"

And then he said, "Sure, we'll let you know," and put the phone down.

Mom had tears in her eyes.

"What happened?" she said.

"He won the first set and was leading 4–2 in the second; then he slipped and fell on the court and after that he couldn't run."

"You mean he hurt his ankle?"

"Bob said his back. He played it out, but lost the third set 6–0."

Mom and Dad were so worried about his back that they didn't even think about David losing; parents are like that. But I cared. It wasn't fair! He *deserved* to win. He was the best, so why couldn't he win?

David called up later to tell us his back was not serious, just a muscle spasm, and he sounded even sadder than I already felt.

"It would have been so easy," he said.

He only had to win two more games.

"Well, congratulations on being the *best* in the United States," I said.

I went down to Roy's house the next day; he invited me to stay overnight and usually we have a ball.

But Dad said no tennis till after my next trip to the clinic, and I had been thinking Roy and I could play in the San Diego Metropolitan doubles, which was the most fun of all the summer tournaments in San Diego.

Roy asked me if I could, the first thing, because the deadline for entering was the next day.

"You better ask somebody else," I said.

"Well, Lutz already called me from L.A. and I said I would if you couldn't."

He didn't even have to call Lutz back. They already had it arranged.

I felt awful. But I couldn't blame Roy. He couldn't sit around just because *I* couldn't play.

Roy has a ping-pong table out in his garage, so we played a while. He isn't as tall as I am, so he has a hard time reaching the short shots; but he scrambles around the table. It looks very funny.

"Let's see how many times we can go without missing," he suggested. We got up to 547 and the ball hit a twig which blew onto the table so we decided not to count that as a miss and we went on. In the 900's I almost missed by stubbing my paddle on the table but I recovered, and at 1065, Roy stubbed his paddle and missed. We saw pingpong balls when they weren't there after that rally!

But I didn't have much heart for pingpong that day. I couldn't stop thinking about David.

"In stories, the best guy always wins," I said. "The guy that keeps trying, and always plays fair, never lost the championship in any story I ever read. *They* don't have bad luck!"

"Those stories aren't very true to life," Roy said. "Some of those writers ought to try playing against a guy that makes bad calls when you don't."

"You said it," I agreed.

Roy's mother asked us what we wanted for lunch, which is a big joke around Roy's house because we always want hamburgers. But even the hamburgers didn't taste any good.

Then after lunch we couldn't think of anything to do, which is the first time that has ever happened to me and Roy. After we sat around for a while, we decided to walk over to the tennis courts at Morley Field, which is not far from Roy's house, and I got to watch him play. Big deal.

I also got to listen to about ninety-nine dozen people say "Too bad David lost! It's a shame!" "How come you're not playing, Johnny?" "You're certainly looking well. Aren't you taking on some weight?"

I didn't want to explode so I walked to the end court where my friend Wilbur gives lessons. He was sitting on the bench waiting for his next pupil, who was late, so I sat down beside him. He didn't say anything about David or why I wasn't playing tennis or the size of my face.

He just said, "Hi, Johnny," and I said "Hi, Wilbur" and we sat there quietly throwing peanuts to a family of ground squirrels who live just outside the fence. They know Wilbur, and will come right up to him and take

the nuts out of his hand. He also has a little bird that is
so fond of him that it hops around on the court even
when he is giving lessons, and it's a wonder nobody ever
steps on it.

Wilbur looks sort of like a hunter in Africa. He has
bright brown eyes and a merry grin, and he wears a
white hat to keep the sun off his head, a gray mustache
to keep the sun off his lips, and long white pants to cover
his wooden leg. He was driving to a tournament one
day when he was a young man, and they had an accident. So instead of being a champion himself, he stands
out in the sun all day throwing balls to little kids. He
must have taught about a million people how to play
tennis.

A lot of them grow up to be champions, like Maureen
Connelly, for instance. A lot more don't even try, but
Wilbur never gets mad; he never raises his voice.

I sat there in the warm sunshine while he gave his
lesson, standing by the net on his good leg, throwing
a basketful of balls out, one by one, to the tall, skinny
boy on the baseline. It was a pretty hot afternoon, and
I got sleepy, watching. I could hear a train in the distance, the Sante Fé, blowing its horn, and those little
bells dingdinging at the crossroads; across the canyon,
in Balboa Park, the carillon chimed four o'clock, and
the animals in the zoo made weird noises.

I could just barely hear Wilbur's voice, I was so drowsy.

"I'd like to have your arm swing out free. Your shoulder
is a big strong one . . ."

"Let the strings do it for you—I don't want those
woody sounds. I want it real smooth."

Cars swished by on Morley Drive, and a plane jetted
in, close overhead.

"Always *want* the ball to go someplace," Wilbur said

patiently. "Then you won't hit all those balls in the net."

"That was a good one. Nice shot."

"Real good."

I must have dozed off because when I looked up there was another pupil, a little Mexican boy about half as high as the net, who was socking the ball with all his might.

"You want to watch this little guy," Wilbur told me. "He's going to be a champion."

"Yeah, if he's lucky," I thought. "If he doesn't hurt his back, or break his leg, or get something horrible wrong with him, that they don't even know what it is."

"Oh, come on, Johnny—you can do better than that!" Wilbur said.

I jerked my head up. But he wasn't talking to me. The little guy's name was Johnny.

"At least I've got both my legs," I thought. "And David can win *next* year."

Wilbur was scooping up tennis balls so I decided to help him. Then I went and rooted for Roy, who was playing singles with a guy about twice as big as he is. Roy is kind of worried because he hasn't started to grow yet. But he didn't have much trouble with the big guy, who ended the match by hitting a ball into orbit.

"Any *other* day he would have beat me," Roy said, with that three-cornered grin of his.

"Yeah, uh'm off m'game," I moaned. "Uh don' know what's the matter with me today. Uh cain't hit a *thang*."

I borrowed Roy's racket and did an imitation of the guy's corkscrew serve, which got Roy laughing so hard that when he'd try to stop he'd burst out again, which cracked me up. I never could stay gloomy very long, especially when I was spending the night with Roy.

4

I Can Play Again

IT ISN'T SUPPOSED TO IN THE DESERT COUNTRY, BUT ONE night late in August it rained all night, and for the first time in three months, I could hear the patter of raindrops, and it sure sounded good.

In the morning I walked around outside and looked at the trees and flowers; you could smell them better since they were wet, and with the dust washed off, the geranium leaves were bright green. The dirt road was spotted with rain, and a rabbit came out from under the cactus, saw me, and froze. The sky had just about cleared up, although there were a few clouds over towards El Cajon.

I decided to play a couple of rounds on the miniature golf course I had built in our backyard when I was eleven—out of bricks, sticks, flower pots, drain tiles, wire screen and an old cement mixer. I could just about play with my eyes shut now that I was fourteen, but the holes were all different and it was still fun. Maybe I could figure out a way to make it tougher, and charge admission.

35

I was just lining up a shot through an old wire bird cage up to the top of a gopher mound when Frank showed up. Frank is my brother-in-law, Frea's husband, and they are building their house on a piece of our hill which Dad and Mom gave them for a wedding present. Frank likes sports of all kinds; he was a football player in high school and he sure looks like it. He's big and blonde, with a butch haircut.

"Would you be interested in a camping trip up to Green Valley Falls?" he asked me.

"Oh boy—would I! When?"

"Soon as you can get ready."

"Who's going?"

"You and me and Frea—Mom says she'll keep the kids."

I thought it was pretty nice of them to take me along, when they didn't have to. Both my brother-in-laws are great guys. Mary's husband, Rol, was in the Air Force and he said he liked to get letters so I wrote him pretty often and he wrote back. Frank and Rol put up a basketball hoop for me and David last Christmas. My dad always intended to, but he never gets around to things like that.

Green Valley Falls is up in the Cuyamaca Mountains, about a forty-five minutes' drive from where we live. We sure are lucky—forty-five minutes east from my house, it is six thousand feet high, and in the winter there's snow and you can go tobogganing. Forty-five minutes' west is the ocean; and even in the winter you can go swimming, if you don't mind getting a little chilly some days.

It was pretty chilly at Green Valley Falls that night. Frank has been camping out all his life but this was my first experience, as my dad is not the hunting and fishing type. We had army cots and sleeping bags—we didn't have a tent—and after a nice day hiking up to the Falls and a delicious supper of sizzling hamburgers, baked potatoes and toasted marshmallows, it all of a sudden got dark—and the temperature dropped to 27 degrees.

We all crawled into our bags, which were fleecelined and very cozy—for awhile. Frea had the cot in the middle with Frank's cot on one side of her and mine on the other, all close together "in case of wild animals," Frea said. I felt rather embarrassed when she said goodnight to Frank—I couldn't help overhearing, naturally. She said, "I love you."

But then she turned over and said, "I love you too, Johnny," so we all burst out laughing.

There weren't any wild animals but it kept getting colder and colder. My sleeping bag turned into an ice box—but if you poked your head out it was even colder outside. At about one A.M. Frea and I made a bolt for the car, where we managed to defrost. Frank was still sleeping peacefully—in his bag.

"He can have it," Frea said. "I don't think we were brought up right, Johnny."

Personally, I thought we were.

But it was an interesting experience, and I wouldn't have missed it.

David was still Back East; after they got his back fixed up he decided to stay and play in the men's tournaments. Dad was afraid he'd have more back trouble, but Mom talked to the doctor long distance and he said it was okay. Also, Dave had won the California State Jaycee Singles so all his expenses were paid.

I was actually looking forward to my next check-up so I could start playing tennis again, but I can't say I enjoyed it much. Dr. Evans decided to perform his favorite operation on me, which he had done a couple of times before. The first thing they do is to put on colored soap which turns my chest a bright orange.

Then they spray on a very cool liquid which is supposed to deaden the skin, but doesn't. Then they stick in a couple of needles and after this they scrape on the bone and take out some marrow.

If your blood is cooling off and chills are racing up your spine, I'll change the subject. If you like the subject, I don't, so I'll change it anyway.

Anyhow, it turned out all right, as Dr. Evans looked at it under the microscope and couldn't find anything wrong with it, so I did get to play tennis after all.

Dad said to begin with I should just play Mom, and Dr. Evans said not to play for twenty-four hours, when I could take the bandage off my chest, so promptly at one o'clock the next day I started playing my first set in almost six weeks, against Mom, and boy was it windy!

We started off pretty close, but I staggered through 6–2. I wasn't playing very well and my smash was as rusty as a fifty-year-old gate that's been rained on twice a week. But Mom gets everything back and you can't beat her unless you're really in there trying, so I felt okay about it. Dad was standing by the net post rooting for me, as usual, but Mom doesn't seem to mind.

"Okay, Dad," I said. "Now it's your turn."

"Tomorrow," Dad said, meaning what he always means when he says "tomorrow"—any time but today. Oh well, there were plenty of guys to play with now that I could play again. I could hardly wait to call Roy. Being restricted to doubles didn't look so bad after a whole summer of not being able to play at all.

The next big tournament coming up was the Pacific Southwest, in Los Angeles, with both adult and junior divisions. It's the week after Forest Hills, the national championships in New York, and David was on his way home.

I called Roy up to tell him I could play doubles again. I figured, when he and Lutz won the San Diego Metropolitan Boys' Doubles, we could win the Pacific Southwest.

"I'm a little rusty," I told him, "but nothing I can't fix up with a couple weeks' practice."

"Well-uh-I didn't know you were going to be able to play," Roy said.

He didn't have to say any more. I knew what he meant. But he could have waited and *asked* me first.

"I'm sorry—I'd rather play with you, Johnny, but . . ."

"That's okay," I said.

Sure, it was okay. Roy could play with Lutz all the rest of his life if he wanted to. I didn't care.

I'd get another partner.

Boy, I felt bad!

David came in on the plane the next day and it was so good to see him that I forgot about Roy until that night, when we were in bed.

"Are you and Roy playing in the Southwest?" he asked me.

"Nope," I said.

"Didn't the doctor say you could play?"

"Yep."

He didn't ask me any more questions, but I guess he found out about it. The next night we were playing bridge, which David had learned how to play when he was back East at the tournaments, and was teaching me how. Mom is a very good bridge player but Dad doesn't care much about it; however, he can play pretty well if he wants to so I naturally didn't expect to win.

Mom explained the point system of bidding to me, and it seemed fairly simple, but Dad says he has more important things to put in his brain so he won't learn it, which Mom says he could in ten minutes if he would listen. But David's bidding was what really drove her wild; he has this "psychological" system—he called it— where he bids the suit that he *hasn't* got. That prevents the person who has got it from bidding it, and then David's partner is supposed to tell what his best suit is, and that is what we play.

We beat Mom and Dad by 3840 to 2210 and Mom said in the future she was going to play something scientific like "Slapjack" or "Steal the Chicken."

Anyhow, we laughed so much that I forgot all about Roy until David said, "Hey, Johnny—how about playing in the *Tribune* Men's Doubles with me in October?"

Me play in the *men's* doubles with *David?* The *Evening Tribune* sponsored the biggest adult tournament in San Diego, and David would probably be top-seeded in singles. He could have anybody he wanted for a partner, And I was only fourteen.

Boy, would Roy be impressed by *that!*

"We'll show 'em," David said, and he wasn't even kidding. He was planning to win.

So was I.

5

Doubles with David

THE ONLY TROUBLE WAS, SUMMER WAS OVER, AND YOU KNOW what that means. *School*.

The year before hadn't been too bad because David was at Granite Hills. He was a Senior and I was a Sophomore, and our tennis team had won the League Championship. Now David was going to UCLA and we didn't have much chance, since most of our other good players had also graduated. Besides, I didn't know anyone very well. It was a big school and I always shot out of there the minute the bell rang.

Most of my friends lived down in San Diego. They thought we were out of our minds to live in "the sticks," and we thought they were out of their minds to live in the city. Of course, Dad and Mom would drive me down to the Morley Field courts to play with them on weekends, and maybe even some days after school. Only I'd have homework.

A few days after school started, my counsellor called me in to her office. In our school district, each class has its own special counsellor who stays with it all four years,

41

but this year we had a new one because the one we had last year got married and quit. I suppose I will get married some day, but I don't know why. I don't even like mixed doubles.

Anyway, this new counsellor was named Mrs. Peterson, so I guess she was already married, and at first I didn't think much of her. She had gray hair, cut short and business-like, and piercing blue eyes, and she didn't believe in fooling around any.

"I see you're good at math," she told me, looking into this big folder with my name on it. "According to these scores you are in the 99th percentile. We've put you in an accelerated group. Can you keep up? How do you happen to be a junior when you are only fourteen?"

I felt like a juvenile delinquent caught robbing a gas station.

"I had to stay out of school a year and I didn't have anything else to do so my Mom taught me a lot of stuff," I admitted.

"Well, it's unfortunate but I suppose there is nothing to be done about it now," she said. "You realize that that is probably why you have these B's on your record instead of all A's."

"Yes, ma'am," I said.

"If you want to get into a good college you'll have to do better this year. With your ability you ought to be able to get a scholarship."

"Yes, ma'am, I'd like to."

"And don't call me 'ma'am'!"

"No'm—Mrs. Peterson."

All of a sudden she grinned at me, and it made her seem much nicer.

"I hear you have a devastating overhead," she said.

I grinned back. She must be a tennis player; nobody else would know what an overhead is.

"About your school activities," she went on, getting back to business. "It is important for scholarship purposes to be a well-rounded individual. I see you already have two varsity letters, but do you do anything besides play tennis?"

"Not much," I admitted.

"Well, why don't you look over this list of school organizations and go out for something else this year? In addition to tennis, of course." Her eyes twinkled.

I looked it over.

"How about the Math Club?" she prodded.

"Yeah—I guess so."

I wasn't too enthusiastic. Math is okay, but I don't like clubs.

"Would you be interested in working on the school paper?"

"No, I wouldn't," I said.

Last year I sent in reports on all the tennis matches, and although my English teacher said I have a flair for sports writing, they didn't get printed. Tennis is a sadly neglected sport, especially in the newspapers. We won our division with twelve wins and two losses, and were not mentioned once in the school paper. We lost all our games in football and basketball, so they said our *track* team was the only bright spot in sports!

"Well—you think about it," Mrs. Peterson said.

It was nice of her to take all that trouble, and I was sorry I'd been so grouchy.

"I will," I promised, "and thanks a lot!"

The next day Mr. Gordon asked us if anybody was interested in playing chess.

My hand shot up a lot faster than it usually does in history class. Quite a few other guys raised their hands, too.

Mr. Gordon said he'd been thinking about starting a chess ladder; the activity schedule was already pretty full, but we could play during lunch periods, and maybe even build up a team to play other high schools.

Boy, would that be neat!

I went up to see Mr. Gordon after class, and the next thing I knew we were sitting in Room 22 with a chess board between us. The only trouble with playing chess at lunch time is, it's over before you know it. At the end of the period I had a four point lead—I won two of his pawns and he sacrificed. I gained another bishop, but lost it in forcing him to trade queens. So I had my castles and a knight and a bishop while he had the same minus a bishop and a pawn. I can tell you right now that game went on for a long time—I finally finished him off after four full periods over a span of four weeks. I used my bishop to get behind his pawns and take them one by one.

Meanwhile we started the chess ladder, and unfortunately they decided to do it alphabetically. Since my name starts with an S I was next to last, and you could only challenge two places above you. However I have to admit that it was worth it, since the first guy I challenged, whose name began with a P, turned out to be my best friend that year. His name was John.

After playing through several lunch periods, he invited me to go home with him one day, and he showed me his collections, which are different from mine, but very interesting. He has rocks, fish, and pigeons. He also collects words—I think. Anyhow he always uses these big jawbreakers. His father was an editor of a newspaper and they had the largest collection of books in the county where they used to live—up near Los Angeles—and I guess he has read just about all of them. He said he would sometimes stay up until 3 or 4 A.M.—*reading*. Boy, are we different!

But I told him about J. R. R. Tolkien, whom I consider the greatest living writer except possibly Charles R. Schulz, the author of *Peanuts,* and he said he had not read *The Hobbit,* so I said I would lend it to him, and he said he would certainly appreciate that.

I never liked to be called "John" myself, but it suited him fine, and since I got to liking him so much I began to like the name too. He was a kind of a short guy, and serious. At school they called him "the absent-minded professor" because he was always forgetting things. One day he left his father's chess set in Room 22 at lunch time and it disappeared and there was a big stink as it was a rather valuable set, so Mr. Gordon made this important rule: quit playing five minutes before the bell rings and put away your set or you will lose your chess pass and not be able to play for a week. I sure hoped nothing like that would happen to me as I had such a long way to get to the top of the ladder.

And John wasn't making it any too easy for me to get past *him*. He was a real brain, but one day I caught him staring off into space so I seized my chance and beat him. He was still dreaming when I packed up the set, sprinted down the hall and challenged my next victim —just as the bell rang.

Meanwhile, the first weekend of the San Diego *Eve-*

ning Tribune Championships had arrived. David was top-seeded in singles, all right, but we weren't seeded in the doubles. There were several good men's teams from San Diego and a team from Los Angeles that was sure to win —everybody said. To be frank, I thought they would myself.

Since we were not seeded, we drew a very tough team in the second round—two of the best men players in La Jolla. I didn't know if we could beat them or not, and we lost the first set 6–3.

But then I noticed that Dave had that determined look on his face, and when he gets that, you better watch out. So I decided to help him win the second set and we did—6–1.

The third set wasn't so easy as they were not surprised any more, and they fought like tigers. But so did David, and he's the best tiger there is. My overhead was going great, because it was so much fun to be playing in a tournament with David, but on set point for us I choked. I popped up a weak volley which they should have murdered—only our opponent also choked, and smashed it into the net; after we shook hands, they had to climb a couple of trees to find his racket!

Somehow I managed to get through the next week—sleeping eight hours every night, doing all my school work, and even downing another guy in chess, where I had worked up to the K's. Our quarter grades came out Friday, and I got two A's and two B's. Some day I am going to get all A's or bust!

Saturday morning I had to go to the clinic, but I wasn't worried. I felt great. I'd been gaining weight, and it was pretty ridiculous to waste all that time and money on a check-up, but that's life.

"Well, I can't find anything wrong with you," Dr. Evans said, after poking around in my stomach and under my arms. I leaped up from the table and started for the door, but had to wait around for a while for the count. Fortunately, they have doubles matches in the afternoon.

Thelma was telling all the doctors and nurses about me being the biggest upset of the men's tournament the week before. She saw it in the paper.

"It's no strain, playing with David," I said. "I only have to cover a quarter of the court."

David was playing the semi-finals of the men's singles at that very moment, and I didn't even get to watch.

"Come on, sweetie, hurry up with that count," Thelma told the nurse at the microscope. "Johnny has to go win another trophy."

"Thanks," I said, "You're a pal."

"Oh, run along," Dr. Evans said. "It's no use your waiting around." Then he told Mom he'd call her, and we zoomed out of there.

David had won his singles in straight sets and we played the number-one team from Pepperdine College in the semis. It was a hot day and I didn't seem to have much pep but David was all over the court, blasting that forehand past them to win 6–3, 6–3.

I resolved to give him a little more help in the finals the next day, especially after the long hot battle he had before he finally won the men's singles.

We were still 10–1 to lose; I was pretty sure we were going to win but I don't bet, unfortunately.

The only thing that worried me was that in late October it gets dark so early that we might not have time to finish, and if we didn't finish, David couldn't play the next weekend because his college team was going some-where, so we would either have to default or flip for the championship, and after all we'd been through I wanted to *win*. Who wants to flip?

You wouldn't think after all the good teams we had beaten that there were any more, but we still had to face the number two seeds, and they were the toughest. The top-seeded team from L.A. had lost in an earlier round.

Although I started out playing well, they broke my serve to forge ahead 2–1, and in doubles all it takes to win a set is one service break. However, I was so mad at myself that I played out of my earlobes and we broke back for 2–2. They got ahead again 5–3, set point, but we held on to make it 5 all. They kept getting ahead, but we refused to lose the set and at 8–8 Dave smiled and said, "Well, we'll just have to outlast them."

We took the next two games and jumped ahead 3–1 in the second set. It began to get dark, and strangely enough no one could hold his serve until Dave finally held at 5–3 for the final game. In five more minutes it would have been too dark to play, and I would have missed the happiest moment of my life.

6

Hallowe'en

THAT WAS THE HALLOWE'EN THAT I WISHED I DIDN'T HAVE
to grow up—the year I was too old to go trick-or-treating
anymore.

We used to have so much fun, scooping out pumpkins
to make jack-o-lanterns, dressing up in home-made cos-
tumes and going up and down the streets ringing door-
bells. We took the biggest paper bags we could find, and
filled them up with candy and apples, and then David
and I would count up to see who got the most. As usual
I was the runner-up.

But the best Hallowe'en I ever had was with Roy, the
year we were eleven. We went to this carnival that his
dad's company was putting on, and Roy was dressed up
like a tramp with baggy pants, a battered felt hat, and a
false nose. I was dressed up like a gypsy, in my sister's
skirt and blouse, with black-yarn braids, and Roy said
I was absolutely bee-yutiful. He and his dad named me
Mabel, and boy, did we have fun at that carnival. We
won a lot of prizes including a large honey-colored bear
that I named Pooh. I won that throwing baseballs at three

milk bottles. When I knocked them all down, Roy said
"Yay, Mabel!" and the caller yelled out, "She's a lady
but she sure throws like a man."

But at the age of fourteen, there I sat in my room,
gloomily staring at Pooh, who looked sympathetic—Pooh
was just like one of the family by then. David was home
for the weekend, but he was out on a date. There was
this girl that only came up to his shoulder and giggled
all the time—girls don't have to be pretty to be popular;
they just have to giggle a lot. But she was pretty too,
worse luck.

Roy had called up, but I wished he hadn't. He wanted
to know if I wanted to go to a *dance*—and I sure didn't.

"Aw, come on, Johnny," Roy said. "What's the matter
with dancing?"

"You have to do it with girls," I muttered.

I guess he thought I was still mad about the doubles,
but I wasn't. What I was really mad about was David.
I'd been looking forward to his coming home for Hallow-
e'en, and then he spent all his time with *her*.

The truth is, I didn't feel very good, but I didn't want
to admit it. I felt kind of tired all the time, but I wasn't
about to mention it and have to go for my check-up any
sooner than I had to. I didn't tackle any tough tennis,
just easy singles and fun doubles.

Roy must have had a good time at the Hallowe'en
dance because whenever I bumped into him at the courts
he was playing mixed doubles. He fixed it up for me to
play with a pretty nice girl who was a good player and
I enjoyed it—until everybody started teasing me about
her. That did it. I decided to concentrate on my chess.
I wanted to get to the top of the ladder by Christmas.

Ironically, I had to play a girl—the only one that came out for chess. She was rather distracting because she talked all the time, but I concentrated hard and managed to win in one and a half lunch periods. She said she heard I was a great tennis star and how come I was so smart, too?

"I mean—athletes aren't usually so smart, are they?" she said. Her name was Laurie.

I'm not so dumb that I believe everything I hear from a girl, so I smiled patiently and assured her that, on the contrary, slow students are not good at athletics any more than they are at anything else, and a lot of the tennis players I know are straight A or anyhow B average students.

"It takes brains to play any sport," I said.

Then Laurie said didn't I think boys were better in math than girls, and I said I didn't know—my sister was pretty good at math, and that made me think of that girl David is so crazy about—she's majoring in *electronics!* You never would know to look at her that she could even do simple arithmetic.

After that Laurie got me to help her with her math homework; and she wasn't kidding, she really couldn't understand it. The bell rang before I could make it clear, so I told her I would finish explaining it after school, if she could meet me in the quad.

She did, and after about ten minutes, she got it! Boy, did I feel good. It's a great feeling when you explain something to somebody and all of a sudden they say, "Oh, *I* get it!"

When my mom came for me, I told her I was just about sure now that I wanted to teach math—of course, if I turned out to be good enough, I'd still like to be on the

Davis Cup, but I seriously doubted if I would ever be that good, unless I could stop getting interrupted all the time.

"You could do both," Mom said.

She thinks I can do anything; you know how mothers are.

About two weeks before Thanksgiving I had worked up to being number eleven on the chess ladder, and I was finally playing Howard, a slippery character who always seemed to be playing someone else when I challenged him. We were concentrating so hard that we didn't notice when it was time to clean up. The bell rang and Mr. Gordon came along and said we should have been cleaned up two minutes before the bell rang. Therefore, he took our passes away for a week. Boy, was I mad. That was a stupid rule.

Mrs. Peterson called me into her office the next day. The Juniors who were going to college had taken the preliminary entrance exams for practice in October, and she told me that I had done well. "How are you coming along in your classes?" she asked.

We were pretty good friends by now, and I said, "How can you get all A's when some teachers don't believe in giving A's?"

"As a matter of record," Mrs. Peterson said, "there are no teachers in this school who never give A's."

Her eyes twinkled, and I had to smile.

"Okay, okay," I said. "I'm working on it."

By the end of that week, the time for my checkup had come and I crossed my fingers. I hadn't been playing much tennis because I just plain didn't feel like it. I knew my red count must be down, and when I walked into the clinic I wasn't too sure when I'd be walking out again.

Thelma was trying to persuade this little guy to let her stick his finger. He was about four years old with blonde curly hair and his bottom lip stuck out about an inch. He was holding his hands tight behind his back, and even his mom couldn't get him to let loose.

"Oh, hi, Johnny," Thelma said. "What a relief! Would you mind showing Richard how we do it?"

I smiled at him and sat down on the stool.

"Be my guest," I said, sticking out one of my fingers.

Richard watched closely while I kept on smiling.

"There now," the nurse said. "That didn't hurt, did it?"

"Sure, it hurt, a little," I said. "Now do I get to look in the microscope?"

They gave me a piece of cotton for my finger and the nurse moved out of my way. I couldn't care less about cells and stuff like that—biology I took because I had to— but the little guy was sure interested. He let them stick his finger and then after his turn at the microscope he and his mom came down the hall and joined us in the waiting room.

"Thank you *so* much," his mother said.

It makes you feel good when people thank you like that, but I never know what to say. I showed the little guy some pictures in a magazine and then we looked out the window at a ship out on the ocean, while our mothers were talking to each other.

"I saw some funny BUGS in that hole," Richard told me.

"So did I!" I grinned at him.

Richard and his mother were gone before Dr. Evans was ready for me.

"What's the matter with him?" I asked my mom.

"He's a little anemic. His mother says he'll be okay."

"Well, that's good," I said. I sure didn't want him to have to be another Wonder Boy.

Finally Dr. Evans called us into his office. Sure enough, my red count was pretty low. He said he didn't know just what to do about it, he'd have to think it over.

"Come back in two weeks," he said.

Two weeks—Hallelujah!

And I thought I'd have to stay there that day.

I was out the front door before they even finished talking. When Mom came out she said we were supposed to call up if I felt any worse so I promised I'd let her know.

But I felt better. Boy, I felt great!

I felt so good that when the phone rang that night and this girl said it was Laurie and would I be interested in this pingpong tournament the recreation center was having during Thanksgiving vacation I said sure, it sounded like fun. I even agreed to play in the mixed doubles with her.

"I didn't even know they *had* mixed doubles in table tennis," I told her.

"Oh, sure. Haven't you ever been in a pingpong tournament?"

"Not in a regular table tennis tournament," I admitted. They have them on the side, sometimes, at tennis tournaments, but that's not like playing against real pingpong players.

"You're supposed to wear black," she said.

I grinned. "That's a switch—in tennis you have to wear all white. You're not even supposed to have any dirt on your shoes."

"Was that a girl?" Mom asked incredulously, when

Laurie finally quit talking long enough for me to hang up without being impolite.

"Yep," I said.

On second thought, there might be problems. How was I going to get to the Recreation Center? I sure as heck didn't want my *mother* to have to drive me and wait around while I played. Laurie had said she'd meet me there, but was I supposed to take her home?

Good grief, I hoped not.

I knew I didn't want to get mixed up with any old girls. Oh well, why worry? It wasn't till Thanksgiving.

Meanwhile, I got my chess pass back, and resumed the game with Howard. After getting two castles behind, I managed to catch up and then made a good pawn move that won a bishop and set up checkmate.

The next day I finished off Grable and went up from ninth to seventh on the ladder. Monday I beat Anderson with a pawn move that opened up a diagonal, making it checkmate. So I was number five!

Tuesday I was playing Benton, number three, and we were exactly even when it was time to put away our sets.

"Hey, Benton," I said. "It's time to quit."

He said, "Don't bother me—I'm thinking." Then he took a long time to make his move. I started picking up the pieces but he was marking down where they were, and I was fidgeting all over the place when Mr. Gordon came up and said, "As this is your second offense, Johnny, I'll have to take that pass for *two* weeks."

I looked at Benton but he didn't say anything, and I couldn't have said anything even if I wanted to be a tattletale. Boy, was I mad!

"What's the matter with *you?*" John asked me in Latin class. "You didn't get annihilated by Benton, did you?"

I told him what happened, and he said it was a gross injustice.

After school Mr. Gordon stopped me in the hall and said that he felt he had been hasty; some of the students had told him of my attempts to warn Benton about the time.

"However," he said. "In the future I'll expect you to be more aggressive. If it happens again, I'll have to take this for the rest of the semester."

And he gave me back my pass. Boy, what a relief.

The next day was the day before Thanksgiving. I had a hard time waking up in the morning and Mom said why didn't I stay home?

I didn't feel very good but I figured it was only one day —and we were having some important tests.

"I better go," I said.

Laurie was in my home room, and she reminded me about the table tennis tournament, Friday night.

I hadn't forgotten. I was looking forward to it. David would be home for the weekend, and he was going to drive me; also he had a neat shortsleeved black jersey he said I could wear with my slacks.

After taking the tests, my head was sort of banging, so I decided not to play chess that day. I had won six straight and climbed from thirteen to fifth place; I had my pass back and could challenge for third again right after Thanksgiving.

"Hey, Johnny!" said this voice close behind me. "I challenge you."

"Oh, no," I groaned.

I turned around and it was Harrison—number seven.

"How about next week?" I said.

"How about today?" he said.

Well, I didn't want to be a slippery character like Howard so I said okay and we sat down with my little travelling chessboard between us.

Harrison made a great attack on my left side, sacrificing a piece and soon regaining it. One of my knights had captured his castle on a king–rook fork. His queen, while attacking my left side, was at the center. Suddenly out of nowhere came his bishop to put me in check. I could do nothing to stop him from checkmating me on the next move. In closely guarding my left side I had left my right side totally exposed. So now I was number *seven*.

"Nice playing," I said.

Boy, it's hard to be a good sport sometimes. I felt more like hurling my chess set out the window.

The trouble was, I knew I had to go home and tell Mom we'd better go to the darn old clinic.

7

Thanksgiving

"A FUNNY THING HAPPENED ON THE WAY TO THE HOSPITAL," Mom told the nurse when we got there. "I fell up the steps and I think I broke my arm."

She was holding onto her left wrist with her right hand, and when she let go, her left hand dangled.

I had been feeling rather dizzy myself on account of my low red count, so I didn't know she had hurt herself when she fell down. Boy, was she brave!

They rushed us to the Emergency Room where we sat and waited about an hour. She told me I'd better go have my check-up, she'd be okay, but I wasn't about to leave her. I wouldn't want everybody to leave *me* at a time like that.

We could hear some doctors in the next room having a cheerful conversation about incisions and scalpels and stuff like that, and Mom said medical jargon was not much like tennis talk, was it?

"Boy, I was really slicing 'em yesterday," I said.

Mom burst out laughing so I kept it up.

"I can't make an incision today, I'm *so* bad," I groaned.

"This scalpel is terrible . . . Man, just three more stitches and I would have had him but I choked."

Mom and I were in stitches ourselves when they came to set her arm. She didn't complain any so I figured the least I could do was not to gripe as usual when it was my turn.

It wasn't much of a surprise to me to find out that my red count had shot down to a new low. They decided to give me a transfusion. Transfusions are great as they make you feel about a hundred per cent stronger in four or five hours, but I can't say I enjoy the five hours. You have to lie absolutely still, with your arm strapped to a board, till you can't tell which is your arm and which is the board. Mom says it only takes about ten minutes to *give* a pint of blood, and she doesn't mind doing it at all, but to get one takes a lot longer because it has to go in slowly. I have this neat stop-watch I got for my birthday, and it comes in handy for timing the drops. It also makes the time pass faster, with those gloomy bells out in the hall going "Pong Pong Pong Pong," so even with your eyes shut you can't help knowing you're in a hospital.

Mom offered to read to me but I didn't feel like bothering to listen. My head was still banging, like when I took the tests—I bet I flunked 'em.

"Boy, that sure was a mistake to go to school today," I thought. "Oh, well—you can't win 'em all."

I cheered myself up by thinking about how nice it was going to be to climb down out of that bed and take off for home. I did it about fifty times—in my head.

Hospital rooms are so horribly *clean*. White curtains, white sheets, white nurses, Mom's arm in a brand new white plaster cast, and me all dressed up in a white—ugh—I refuse to call it by name. My room at home has red and blue wall paper with prancing horses, and flower-pots and peasant boys and girls waving their hands; and I have a blue rug, and blue and white curtains, and a whole set of rubber Charlie Brown characters—Peanuts, Lucy, Linus, Snoopy and Charlie Brown's little sister Sally —all grinning down at me from the top of my bureau. Man, is it cheerful!

I was almost going to sleep when I heard somebody outside the screen that we had blocking the door so we could have plenty of fresh air without losing our privacy.

"I don't think you'd better come in right now," was a nurse's voice, I think, and then this man's voice said, "But he's on the critical list . . ."

It broke off, like somebody said "Sssh!" and my mom streaked out of the room in no seconds flat. A few minutes later she came back looking very mad.

"Hey, Mom," I said, "What's all this about me being on the critical list?"

"Weren't . . . you asleep?" Mom asked. I knew she was trying to figure out something to say that wouldn't be a lie. She wouldn't lie to me.

"Am I?" I demanded.

"Well, you have been before," she said. "And you got all right again. It's automatic when your blood count is low, Dr. Evans said. It doesn't mean anything."

"You're darn right it doesn't!" I said. "I'm not about to die, that's for sure."

I never saw my mom look so mad. She was about to bust.

I was pretty mad myself.

"How ridiculous can they get?" I muttered.

Sure enough, we were right, and I didn't. But Dr. Evans

said I had to stay in the hospital and have another transfusion the next day.

"Oh, no," I said. "It's *Thanksgiving!*"

Thanksgiving dinner in a hospital—brother!

The dietitian came up from the kitchen to ask me what I wanted—how would I like some nice creamed turkey? (Did you ever notice that even the *food* in a hospital is white?)

"I'll have a drumstick," I said.

The dietitian, who was quite young and pretty, burst out laughing.

"Okay," she said. "I'll get you a drumstick if I have to cook the turkey myself."

"Don't worry," Mom told her. "We'll bring him one from home."

"Hey," I said, rather alarmed. "You're going to stay with me, aren't you?"

She always did. The first night she slept on three chairs pushed up together. After that they brought her a cot.

"Of course," she said. "Frea's cooking the dinner anyway."

So Mom stayed, and we had a pretty good Thanksgiving dinner. After my second transfusion I was starved, and it sure tasted great, even in those dismal surroundings. Of course, I missed all the little kids. Our family was getting pretty big now. Frea had all Frank's folks as well as all of ours to dinner, and they had to use the pingpong table, there were so many.

My sister Mary came to see me during visiting hours. She is the only one in our family who isn't tall, but she about made up for it in circumference, as she was about to have a baby any minute. Just the same she looked very cute. Some people call her "Red" because of her hair, but it's really not much redder than mine and Frea's; everybody calls Frea "Sandy," and I have been referred to in the sports pages as a "Strawberry blonde," but you know how sportswriters are. Anything for a different word. I sure wish they hadn't thought of *that* one!

Mary brought me the latest "Peanuts" book and asked me if I would be her baby's godfather.

Gee. Me a godfather. That was even better than an uncle.

But maybe I shouldn't.

I asked Mom if she would get me a drink of pop, and hoped she wouldn't figure out that I was doing it to get rid of her. As soon as she was out of the room I said, "The only thing is, I'm supposed to see that it gets brought up right—right?"

Mary said she was sure I would, that's why she wanted me to be the godfather.

"Well, I was on the critical list," I told her. "I don't figure on dying, but I just thought you ought to know."

Mary looked awfully serious. "I don't figure on it either but—if you did, Johnny, then you'd be the best godfather she could possibly have."

I thought about that. Gee, that was a nice thing for her to say.

We smiled at each other. "Okay, then," I said. "And thanks a lot."

When Mom came back we told her I was going to be Christy's godfather.

"Christy?" Mom said, looking quizzically at Mary's middle.

"Christine Mary," Mary said.

"You're sure about that?"

"They already have two boys," I explained.

The next day was the day of the table tennis tournament, and Dr. Evans wouldn't let me go home. I was feeling so good I could have played, except that I couldn't use my right arm, and I'm not too good at doing things lefthanded. I couldn't straighten my arm yet because of a bruised vein, but it was nothing serious.

"What about Laurie?" I asked Mom.

"Well—you'd better call her. Just tell her where you are," Mom said. "She'll understand."

They had a telephone right next to my bed, so I couldn't get out of it. It was the first time I ever called up a girl. I had to ask this character that sounded about ten years old if I could speak to her.

"Hey, Laurie," he sang out. "It's a boy! It's a different one, I think . . ."

There was a lot of shushing and a scuffling sound, and then Laurie said, "Hello?"

"This is Johnny," I said.

"Oh, Johnny! I'm so glad you called. Did you have a nice Thanksgiving?"

"Well, it was unusual," I said. "I'm in the hospital."

"The hospital?" she said. "Oh, *Johnny*."

"So I can't go."

That was putting it bluntly, but it was the first time I ever broke a date. As a matter of fact, it was the first time I ever had a date.

"Oh, I'm *so* sorry," Laurie said.

"I'm sorry too—well, goodbye," I said, and hung up. Thank goodness that was over.

I had to stay in the hospital ten days. Mom shouldn't have been waiting on me with a broken arm, but with my right arm out of commission, we only had two good hands between us. So she helped me, and I helped her, and we got along great. The nurses said we were no trouble at all.

But I sure hoped that next time they would ruin my *left* arm!

Next time, I thought. What was the matter with me? Was I getting resigned to my fate? Dr. Evans was trying a new kind of medicine—this time it was going to work. It ought to; it cost twenty-two cents a pill! At three pills a day, that was more than a brand new tennis ball.

But at least these new pills didn't blow up my face. It would be nice to look like myself for a change. And I felt like myself, too, thanks to whoever donated the necessary corpuscles.

Dr. Evans let me out of the hospital the first Saturday in December, and by that time Mary was already out of another hospital with her baby, which she had right after she left me on Thanksgiving!

Sure enough, it was Christine Mary, and we were going to call her Christy.

Boy, she was little. She was all done up in a pink blanket, but Mary opened it up and let me look at her hands and feet. She had all the right number of everything, but her fingernails were only as big as the head of a pin.

She was very pretty, with soft white skin and just a little bit of hair that curled over on top of her head, and she was so fat she had dimples—all over.

My sisters had had babies before, but I never paid that much attention when they were brand new. That was because I never was a godfather before.

Not long after I got out of the hospital we stood up in the chapel, by the baptismal font, with a bunch of other godparents and their babies, and I had to hold her. The

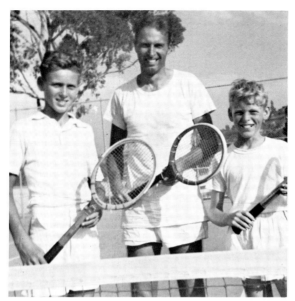

David, George (Johnny's father), and Johnny (at age 10).

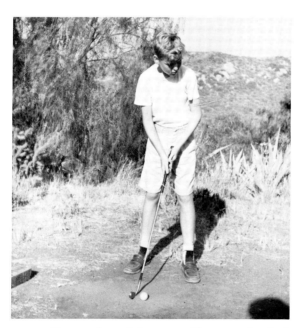

Johnny, age 11, on the miniature golf course he had made himself.

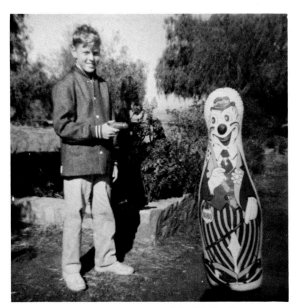

Johnny, age 11, with "Bobo."

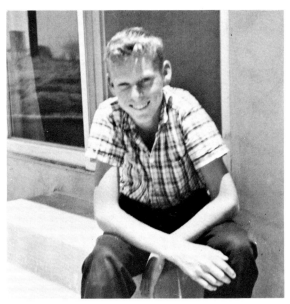

Johnny at age 14.

parents are not very important at a christening—they just stand back and watch. Some of the babies cried, but Christy didn't. I could say she was a little angel, or a cherub, or something, but to tell the truth, she was asleep.

Boy, that was a happy day. You don't appreciate how good it is to have a home till you get to go home to it from the hospital. My room looked just as cheerful as ever, with Charlie Brown beaming down at me from the top of my bureau, and Pooh sitting studiously at my desk.

I was whistling over my penny collection, which was now worth $20.57 (I turn it in in penny rolls for dollar bills, but I keep count) and my mom stuck her head in the door.

"Hey, Mom," I said. "You shouldn't be so generous. Guess how many pennies I've wangled out of you and Dad in the past three years?"

"Hundreds, I guess," she admitted.

"Over two thousand."

"Wow."

She sat on my bed and we talked a while; then she said, "What do you want for Christmas?"

"Golly," I said. "I don't know." Boy, was I glad I wasn't going to be in the hospital for *Christmas!*

8

Christmas

TELLSON'S, MY HOME LOAN OFFICE, WAS ALWAYS BESIEGED around Christmas time. Everybody wanted money to buy presents. The only trouble was, I needed the money myself, for the same reason.

However, my finances were in pretty good shape that year. I had $17.21 saved up from my clothes allowance, $33.74 from my regular allowance, $20.57 in my penny collection, and $44.60 in capital, from miscellaneous stuff like racket-carving, running ads in *The Spy*, babysitting, etc. I'd rather save money than spend it—except at Christmas. It's an awful temptation when you are an uncle.

I got the Christmas spirit pretty bad. I didn't want to be like Scrooge, so I decided to lower my interest rates and give out a stick of chewing gum with each loan. I also offered my services to Mom as a Sanitary Engineer (i.e., taking out the garbage) FREE and advertised pencil sharpening, no charge, on the new sharpener Dad put up on my bureau, when I had been planning on charging for that.

But that was nothing to what happened to me when I got turned loose in the toy department.

"Remember when I got Bobo for Christmas?" I asked Mom. Bobo was a big rubber clown with weights in his bottom, who was about as tall as I was when I was eleven years old. He was for punching and boy, did I ever give him a licking. I was pretty skinny that year and I was building myself up. He was my favorite present.

When you are fourteen years old, you can't ask for toys any more, but you wish you could because there's nothing else you really want. Being an uncle is the perfect solution.

I got a musical rocking chair for Bryan, who turns on whenever he hears music; a huge Panda for Craig; a small table and chair set with toy dishes for Kathy, who is always helping her mother with the housework; a rocking horse for Teri; and a baby swing for Christy. Mom and I were still pooling our two good arms as her left was still in the cast and my right was still unbendable, although improving.

We both spent a whole bunch of money on Frea and Frank and Mary and Rol, who had these long lists of stuff they needed for their houses—like towels, for gosh sake—I guess that's what happens when you get married. It was hard to figure out what to give David but he needed a new bicycle tire for riding his bike around college so I decided to give him that and I gave Mom a game and my father a book. Mom and I always give each other games for Christmas. Once we gave each other the same one!

I also made a list of what I wanted, and put it in *The Spy*, Vol. I, #18, Sunday, Dec. 10, 1961.

Wanted for Christmas

Small safe
Post cards from other states (available by mailing to
    Chamber of Commerce)
Socks
Folders
Subscription to *Peanuts*
Globe of the world
Typewriter
Pens (blue) Lindy ball point
Good compass
Cushion
Chair
Bathrobe

That was all I could think of. Naturally, I didn't expect
to get the typewriter, but they said to put down everything I wanted, so I did. It would be nice for typing my
newspaper instead of printing it all by hand. And also, I
would like to learn to type—I could type my school papers and maybe get better marks.

The more I thought about it, the more I wanted that
typewriter. If they hadn't insisted on me making a list, I
probably never would have even thought of it.

Meanwhile, I had to get my mind off Christmas for a
while and do some homework. My parents had decided
I shouldn't go back to school until after the vacation, so
I was doing my work at home. Mrs. Peterson got my assignments together and Dad picked them up.

I planned my homework schedule on Wednesday and
plunged in Thursday. In three days I read a book, made
a report, and did about half my algebra. Then I took care
of history, my Latin report, Hamlet, a composition for

English, and read Benjamin Franklin's autobiography. I translated one story in Latin every night, but didn't do any work on Sundays. There are some advantages to doing your work at home, and some disadvantages. I sure hoped it wasn't going to wreck my grades.

John Parsons came over to see me the first day of vacation. We were playing a game of chess when he said, "Oh by the way, Johnny, there was something I was supposed to bring you but I forget what."

I kept on trying to find out whenever he came over, but I never found out till I went back to school. It was a Christmas card which all the kids in my class had signed. And he forgot and left it in the chemistry lab.

"Poor old absent minded professor," I said, shaking my head.

I also spent the weekend before Christmas with Roy and polished up my pingpong, since Laurie had called up to tell me there was another tournament at the recreation center on the 23rd of December. Fortunately my arm was back in business so I said I would play in it.

Frea and Frank went up to the mountains and brought back some mistletoe. David and Dad and I picked out the tree—a beauty! Christmas cards began piling up, and we all went around singing Christmas carols. I think Christmas carols are by far the best kind of music. Rock and roll is just a whole lot of noise, yelling and confusion. Christmas carols are sometimes sentimental, but they are happy, not sad. The writers of these songs must have been inspired by the season. Classical music can be pretty good, but there is something in a Christmas carol that no other type of music has. It is hard to put into words, but it is there.

Every year since I can remember we have had a

Christmas carol party on Christmas Eve, singing carols and having punch and cookies. All the neighbors used to come, but when we moved to the country we didn't have many neighbors and besides our family was having a population explosion so we just about filled up the living room ourselves.

This year, though, Mom was so excited about getting the cast taken off her arm, two days before Christmas, that she forgot all about the party, and I wasn't any help in reminding her, because of the table tennis tournament.

David said he would drive me to the recreation center, so Mom wouldn't have to, but he took Arnell along. They weren't engaged yet, but they were just about inseparable —they had sweaters just alike, and they went around holding hands all the time. Boy, that sure was a surprise to me. David holding hands with a girl!

Arnell said I looked very nice in David's black jersey and black slacks; I wasn't as tall as David yet, but I was on the way, and I was taller than Arnell. Laurie was pretty tall, too, and when David saw her he said, "Wow— she's a blonde!"

"Knock it off, will you?" I muttered.

She was wearing this black outfit that fit all over and I was pretty embarrassed, until we got started playing. There was just this big room full of pingpong tables and boy, was it fun.

They had the singles first and much to my surprise I won the Boys Fifteen and Under. David played in the Eighteens and got knocked out in the second round. I guess the older guys must have been pretty tough because I have never won a game from David.

Arnell just watched in the singles, because David is only beginning to teach her how to play, but when it came to the mixed doubles, which were not divided into age groups, she played with David, and Laurie and I drew them in the first round, worse luck.

"I never beat David at anything," I told Laurie.

"Well, you're about to," she said, smiling up at my brother.

She and Arnell both giggled all over the place, but David and I were in dead earnest. You could see that he wasn't about to let his kid brother beat his best girl.

Laurie was pretty shook when he fired that patented unreturnable serve at her, and when he started walloping forehands all over the place the outlook was pretty bleak.

My usual steady, relaxed game which had managed to overcome the Fifteen and unders was duck soup to David, and since in pingpong doubles you have to take turns returning the ball, my only chance was to overwhelm Arnell when it was her turn.

After a seesaw battle up to 20-all, I hit the ball as hard as I could at Arnell, and it just missed the edge of the table by a hair. David won the next point and the game, by *not* missing the edge of the table in front of Laurie.

I turned to Laurie to apologize but she had her lip stuck out a mile.

"You can *too* beat your brother," she said, flinging back her hair. "Come *on*, let's go!" It was the best two out of three games.

The second game was just as close, but on the last point, with Laurie yelling, "Come on, Johnny!" I fielded one of David's fiercest shots from halfway across the room, and my return just rolled over the net and died.

Dave might have been able to reach it, with his long arms, but it was Arnell's turn and she would have had to crawl across the table to get it.

After that, we mopped up on the third game, 21–15. Laurie was jumping up and down, screaming, and I grinned at David, who was looking sort of crestfallen.

"It's not much like tennis," I said. In tennis, you're not supposed to make any noise, but I don't know why not. It was kind of exciting.

"Nice going," Arnell said, sincerely. "I'm glad you won, Johnny."

"Gee," I said, "Thanks, Arnell. Thanks a lot." And David grinned at me, too.

After that, I couldn't lose. Laurie and I won the mixed doubles.

So I went home from my first table tennis tournament with two trophies! How do you like that?

The next day was Christmas Eve, and in the middle of the afternoon we were busy wrapping presents when Mom put her fingers up to her mouth and said, "Oh my goodness, I forgot! For the first time in twenty years—I forgot our carol party."

"Why don't we call everybody up right now?" I said.

"Oh, I'm afraid it's too late. They'll all be doing something else, and I haven't got the stuff for the punch—oh dear."

Mom was terribly disappointed, and so was I.

"Well, you and I and Dad can sing," I said.

So Dad came in from his typewriter and sat down at the piano and we started singing "Joy to the World!" Carols ought to have more people but we were doing okay when David came in with Arnell and they joined in.

Then Frea and Frank came up the hill with Kathy and Teri, and Mom said, "I'd better call Mary and Rol—just in case they can still come."

"Oh, *they're* coming," Frank said cheerfully. "Rol was the one that reminded me—'we always sing carols at Mom's house on Christmas Eve.'"

So everybody came, and we had peanut butter sandwiches and pop and Christmas cookies, and we had the best carol party we have ever had.

The minute Dad touched the piano keys, Bryan started dancing around the room. Kathy was hanging over Baby Christy saying, "Oh, she is such a *tiny* baby. We have to be *careful* of her—isn't she *beautiful?*" Teri was lifting her arms up to everybody to be picked up and hugged, and Craig was just sitting on the floor, staring at the Christmas tree with big round eyes.

After they left, Mom and Dad and I sat in the living room with the Christmas tree lights, all colors, reflected in the shiny black windows. It was very quiet and peaceful; we didn't talk.

Happiness is not what you feel when you get everything you want, because I felt that way the next morning, when I got my typewriter.

Happiness is the way you feel when you sing "Silent night, Holy night" and "Joy to the World" and then just sit in the darkness and think about it.

9

Berkeley

NEXT TO SAN DIEGO COUNTY, I GUESS I LIKE SAN FRANCISCO. They have a neat newspaper, *The Chronicle,* and my favorite baseball team, the Giants. On my various trips up to Berkeley to see the doctors at the University of California, I've seen just about all the sights—Chinatown, the Golden Gate Bridge, Fisherman's Wharf and so on. We rode on a cable car, which is very exciting when you are only eleven years old, which I was the first time I did it. It's a trolley car with no sides so you sit on these open benches and hang on for dear life as you go down the steepest hills any vehicle I know of has ever negotiated— also around these hair-raising curves, all the time clang-clanging and the driver putting on the brakes. Boy, what if they slipped! You'd find yourself in a heap at the bottom.

We also took the Harbor Cruise and saw the island of Alcatraz, which is very grim and desolate looking, although not very far from civilization. I didn't think they ought to keep people in a place like that, and now they don't anymore. We had steak at this famous steak place where they cook it over the open fire while you wait, and it isn't too expensive. I'd rather eat steak than anything you could name, and since my father has this policy of building me up, I get to have it pretty often.

I was kind of surprised when my parents told me we were going up to Berkeley a couple days after Christmas. My red count was pretty good again and I had gained over twenty pounds in four weeks, which is some kind of a record! Even babies don't do that well, although my sisters were always bragging about theirs. Besides, Dr. Evans wanted me for another exhibition as one of his "prize patients," in the spring.

My mother explained there had been some "new developments" at the Donner Laboratory up at the University and they wanted to make some tests. Well, I sure as heck didn't want to have my school work interrupted again, not to mention having to quit playing tennis all the time; so I said okay, let's go, and get it over with during the vacation. Dr. Evans also agreed, although he was always grumbling about our going off on these "wild goose chases." Mom explained that the difference was, Dr. Evans was a top hematologist (that's a specialist in blood diseases) but he was working on controlling whatever was wrong with me, through drugs, and he was doing a great job of it, but the doctors and scientists at Berkeley were also working on a cure.

I've always enjoyed taking trips. You wake up in the middle of the night, or anyhow when it's still dark, and your dad says, "We're leaving in ten minutes!" Ordinarily I don't like to get up early, but on a trip it's different— it's exciting, driving along the empty freeways, with the sky getting lighter and lighter, and then the sun coming up, so you can get through L.A. before the morning rush.

That morning it was foggy along the coast, and before daylight you couldn't see where you were going, but Dad got behind a big truck, which was outlined in red lights, and followed it. We weren't quite sure it was going to Los Angeles, but we hoped so, and it was.

We had our second breakfast at a pancake house north of L.A.—Dad always orders pigs in a blanket, which is hot cakes wrapped around sausages, and Mom gets a Denver omelette, but I prefer good old ham and eggs, sunny side up, with pancakes on the side. They had six different kinds of syrup but I like plain maple; that boysenberry stuff reminds me of something you'd turn up under a rock. When I said that, Mom said she would never be able to eat it again, and switched to honey.

"And please don't make any remarks about *honey!*" she shuddered.

Half the fun of a trip is the places you eat, and stopping at motels. Motels are much more fun to stay at than hotels; they have a friendly atmosphere, while hotels have a stuffed shirt type of atmosphere. The one we stayed at that night had very comfortable beds, free TV, and a swimming pool, which Mom and I were the only ones to patronize. Dad stood on the balcony of the motel, watching us, and agreeing with all the other guests who passed by and said we must be some kind of nuts. But it was a heated swimming pool! What the heck did they think it was for?

About the middle of the second day we arrived in Berkeley, and after finding a motel went straight up to the campus of the University of California. The Donner Lab is at the back end of the campus so we drove through, and boy, is it busy even during vacation. They had quite a few students with long hair and weird clothes—I believe San Francisco is where the beatniks first got started, and then they spread, but there were more of them at Berkeley than I have seen at any other college. There were also more bookstores in the town than I have ever seen anywhere else.

The Donner laboratory is, of course, a place for research, but they also have a clinic that reminded me too clearly of the one back home. They do all the same things to you.

"No wonder I don't have enough blood when you keep taking it out of me!" I joked.

But I like the doctors up there very much, and they seem to like me. That day I met a new one, Dr. Vogel, and boy, was I surprised? She was a lady!

She was fairly young, with short dark hair and blue eyes. She wore one of those starched white coats the doctors wear and her hair was very neat, but still it looked nice, and she was just about as tall as I was. But what I liked about her more than any other doctor I ever had was that she was so gentle.

The other ones poke around in your ribs like you're a sack of potatoes. And even the nurses can be pretty rough when they are getting a sample of what's inside of you. I suppose they get so used to it that they don't think that the poor patient might not be as used to it as they are. Personally, I never did get used to it, and I never will.

Anyway, Dr. Vogel was different. She noticed right away that my right arm was still bruised, and she told the nurse who usually does it that she would take the sample herself. Then she was as careful as she could be, and when I said, "Ouch!" she said, "Oh, Johnny, I'm sorry."

"That's okay," I said. "I shouldn't gripe so much."

Nobody ever apologized to me before; usually they say, "Oh, now, *that* didn't hurt."

Ha, ha.

"Thanks for using my left arm," I said. "I've got a tournament coming up."

"I wish you'd tell me how to keep score," she said. "There are some courts right up the hill from here and some of us have been learning how to play but we always get mixed up . . ."

"Oh, I'd be very happy to," I said. I love to teach people things. I even taught my grandmother how to keep score in tennis.

"We had a big argument over whether the first point is five or fifteen." She sat down on the stool as if she had plenty of time to talk to me.

"Some people call it five or fifth, and some call it fifteen, but it's the same thing, not both. Fifteen is correct. Then comes thirty, forty, and game."

"What about deuce?" she asked.

"That's when it's a tie; you always have to be two points ahead of your opponent in order to win a game. So when it's forty-all they call it deuce, and you have to get two points in a row in order to win. If you win one point, it is called your 'ad,' or advantage. Then if you win the next point, it is game, but if you lose it, you go back to deuce."

She got out a little notebook and wrote it down.

"That's very clear," she said. "Maybe you can give me some other pointers sometime."

"I'd be glad to," I said.

After that I met a little boy out in the hall, who was the first person they had ever tried out this new development on. He was about the age of Richard, but he had dark hair and rosy cheeks.

"Stick em up!" he said, drawing two guns out of the holsters on his belt, so I stuck 'em up.

I didn't understand just what it was they tried out on

him, but whatever it was, he looked pretty healthy and Mom said maybe we could come back next summer and do it.

I wasn't too enthusiastic, but summer was a long way off. Why worry?

On the way back to San Diego, Mom suggested that we stop and see Hearst Castle, which we had never seen. I said, "No thanks." She also mentioned picking up a few shells on Shell Beach, but I said, "No thanks." Santa Claus, California, is a place where you can mail postcards and stuff with a Santa Claus postmark, and they have stores where you can buy toys and souvenirs, but I was in too much of a hurry. The only thing Mom got to do was eat some famous pea soup at Andersen's.

When we crossed the San Diego County line, green fields turned to sagebrush, but it sure looked good to me. Boy, did it feel good to get home!

We have this neat book called *The Fireside Book of Folk Songs* which we sing out of sometimes. It has a lot of jolly songs like "Oh my Darlin' Clementine" and "Doodah" and "Jimmie Crack Corn an' I don' Care" and "I Been Wukkin' on de Railroad." But my favorite is

When Johnny comes marching home again, hurrah, hurrah!
We'll give him a hearty welcome then, hurrah, hurrah!
The men will cheer, the boys will shout,
The ladies they will all turn out,
And we'll all
Feel
Gay
When
Johnny-comes-marching-home!

10

Varsity

WITH DAVID AND TWO OTHER GOOD SENIORS GONE TO college, the prospects of our tennis team winning the League Championship were not too good. I was number one, our number two and three men—George and Dennis —were good players, but after that you could take your pick of all the guys who came out for tennis. My friend John, who was on the Jayvees last year, was very anxious to make the team, and we worked out every day after school. He worked like a beaver, but let's face it, he was not as good as he wanted to be.

"I'm about as coordinated as a plaid jacket and striped pants," he grumbled.

"My mom isn't very coordinated, but she's pretty good," I encouraged him. "She can beat my brother-in-law who was a football star in high school—it just takes practice."

So we practiced. Unfortunately, John didn't have twenty years to develop, like Mom did. He just had a couple more weeks before Coach chose this year's Varsity.

I heard rumors about the new Senior, Dick Kendale,

who had just transferred from the East, before I ever met
him. Everybody said he was great. Coach told me that
with him we might be able to win after all. We needed
just one more good man.

Coach was a little short guy with curly brown hair and
the most energy I ever saw in one person. At our matches
he was all over the place, bouncing around and urging
us on to victory. It's kind of hard to get used to high
school tennis after you play tournaments because in tournaments everybody maintains this deathly silence, but in
high school everybody is screaming and yelling. I think
if they would permit more rooting at the big tournaments instead of shushing everybody up, tennis might
become a more popular sport. However, it *is* hard to concentrate sometimes, when the championship of your
school is riding on one well-placed smash—and somebody
in the stands sings out, "Miss it!"

That would never happen at Forest Hills.

Anyhow, I was looking forward to playing this new
guy. From all I heard, I figured he might be number one,
but I wasn't going to give up my spot without a struggle.
I figured he might come under the heading of "easy
singles," and if not, I could concede if I *had* to.

Came the day when he was all squared away in our
gym class, and out he trotted across the field to the
courts. We have sixteen courts at our school, which is
only two years old, but whoever built them was no tennis
player. There was nothing to stop the wind, the sun was
in your eyes, they were all marked up with different
colored lines besides the tennis lines—multi-purpose
courts, these are called, so you can play basketball, volley-
ball, etc., but it sure is confusing when you are playing

tennis. I'd rather have half as many tennis courts and put the basketball backboards somewhere else. Of course, we kidded a lot about making a basket on set point, or getting crosseyed trying to decide whether a shot was in or out, with all those lines; however, we were used to it.

But poor old Kendale! He just stood there bugeyed, with his hands on his hips, looking around.

"You call these tennis courts?" he asked.

He was a very big guy, with a brown crewcut. I'm getting tall, but he made me look like a shrimp. And with my phenomenal gains in weight—I was almost up to 140 —I wouldn't call myself skinny. But Kendale was huge. He must have weighed over 200.

When Coach introduced us, I couldn't help thinking of the referee at a prizefight, and my hunch didn't prove too wrong. I could tell from the start that Kendale didn't care much for me, and to tell the truth I wasn't too impressed with him.

"This your number one player?" he asked Coach.

"Yep," I said.

He gave the air a couple of vicious swipes with his racket—a backhand and a forehand, in that order. Then he raised it a couple miles over his right shoulder and brought it crashing down past his left knee. This is called an American Twist.

"Kendale has been number one on his team in New Jersey for the past three years," Coach told me. "I guess you'd better play him a set, Johnny."

"Oh, sure," I said. "I'd be glad to."

After we had warmed up for fifteen minutes, I asked him if he was ready to play. I figured the gym period would be over before we got started. He didn't exactly say no, so we started.

He measured the net. He said he hadn't played in three months, and that he'd been up pretty late last night—but he seemed fairly confident. The other guys were supposed to be practicing, but I don't think any of them were keeping their eye on the ball that day. And Coach was right there on the sidelines taking it all in.

It wasn't much of a set. I beat him 6–0. I could have given him a couple of games to make him feel better except that I learned the hard way, in the Eleven and unders, that that can be suicide. Of course, I could have let him off the hook if he hadn't been such a good player, but he *was* good.

I went up to the net to shake hands, since we didn't have time to play another set.

"Nice playing," I said. "We sure can use you on the team."

I guess I must have sounded patronizing but I sure didn't mean to. I didn't know what else to say.

He was pretty mad. He said I didn't let him warm up long enough. The court had a bad glare; he was used to playing on Lay Kold; the slant in the court bothered his overheads; and didn't anybody ever hear of a windbreak out here?

I could see his point—I was playing on home ground, and I was all ready to say I'd be glad to play him again when he said, "Besides, with these crazy lines you can call the ball any old way you want to."

I got hot all over. Boy was I furious!

"I am *not* noted for my cheating," I said, and aimed for the gym, walking as fast as I could walk.

I got a lot of sympathy from the other guys. Nobody liked Kendale.

"He's a sorehead," George said, after playing him for

the number two spot, and winning in two close sets. Dennis eked out his number three spot with an after-school match that lasted until dark—Dennis won 10–8 in the third. So I didn't have to play him again, and Kendale was number four.

Coach went around with this corrugated frown under his curly brown hair.

"What am I going to do about doubles?" he asked me one day. "George and Dennis both want to play with you."

I was the captain of the team, and in the "bush league" as we call the county high schools, strategy counts a lot. Each team has four men who play singles, and four others who play doubles. Each singles player plays one set with each of the singles players on the opposing team, winning one point for each set he wins, so the most he can win is four points. But the two doubles teams play each other, and for each win they get four points—or a total of eight. Therefore most of the schools have their best players play doubles, since a strong player can often "carry" a weaker one, and win twice as many points.

Kendale wanted to play singles anyway, so we decided to let him try it.

"George and Dennis could play doubles together," I suggested to Coach. "And what about me playing with John, if he makes the team?"

The year before, my brother had won all his matches with the number eight man as his partner, so maybe I could—and besides, John and I knew each other pretty well. I could get us some practice matches and we could work out a good strategy.

The only trouble with this plan was that it didn't work out very well.

Our first match was with the weakest school in the

league, and we should have beaten them decisively, but we just barely grazed by them.

George and Dennis turned out to be a great team, and won their eight points, but John was so excited at the prospect of playing doubles with me that he couldn't hit a thing when he was playing his challenge match for the number eight spot on the team—so he lost and I had to play with this other fellow I hardly knew. Actually he wasn't as good as John, but that's the way the ball bounces. John would be allowed to challenge him again, though, and I wished him better luck next time.

Anyway, Green and I won one of our doubles matches but lost the other, so we gained only four points instead of eight. Kendale won three out of four singles, and two other guys on our team won one singles match apiece, so we beat our opponents by the narrow margin of 17–15. And our next match was with a much tougher school.

Things looked pretty black, and on top of that the morale on our team was terrible. Kendale kept threatening to quit—nobody liked him and he knew it.

It was up to me to do something about it, I finally realized. With four good players we ought to be able to win the championship. We could win all the doubles for sixteen points, and count on just *one* of our singles players coming through on one match, at the very least, for the point that would break the tie.

The more I thought about it, the more I knew what I had to do, and I don't mind saying I was chilled at the prospect. I would have to ask Kendale to be my doubles partner.

Good grief.

Unfortunately, when you decide to get along with somebody, the guy doesn't always agree—so when I walked up to Kendale and asked him how about us playing doubles together in the next Varsity match, he glared at me.

I swallowed my pride a couple of times and tried again. "How about a practice match against George and Dennis?" I said.

He knocked his racket against the net cord a couple times and then said okay. I'm afraid he was chiefly motivated by a burning desire to beat George and Dennis, and they didn't look too happy when I broke the news to them, but I tried to get the point across that it was for the good of the team.

George is a tall skinny darkhaired guy who wears glasses, and Dennis is stocky, with sun-bleached hair, and a nose with the top layer of skin peeled off.

It was a terrific match. I really enjoyed it. We all played out of our ear lobes and the points were fast and furious. But Kendale and I lost.

This was not what Kendale had in mind, and he started griping again. He hadn't been expecting to play today; he wasn't in shape; and if I hadn't lost my serve we would have won the match . . .

I blew my top. "I can't win my serve if you hit all your volleys into the net," I said. "And I can't help it if you don't keep yourself in shape, and I can think of a lot of people I'd rather have for a partner! I like to have *fun* when I play tennis!"

Then I stalked off.

In the locker room everybody was sympathizing with me again and nobody would say a word to Kendale. He was sitting on a bench, all by himself, taking off his tennis shoes.

I stood it as long as I could. These were all my friends,

and he was a new guy. Back East he was used to being number one, and I wouldn't like it if I was top man on my team for three years and then had to be number four when I was a senior.

I went over. "Hey, Kendale," I said. "I'm not looking for enemies. I think we'd make a great doubles team, and we'll beat 'em next time."

He looked up. There was a funny expression on his face. I couldn't figure it out.

Then he said, "Cheese—you really mean that, don't you?"

"Sure," I said.

He shook his head.

If I was waiting for an answer, I didn't get it that day, but after that we were friends. I found out that his folks had broken up—they were trying to wait till he got through high school but they had this big explosion on Christmas Day and his mom took off for California, taking him with her.

He didn't want to go.

"Well, maybe you'll get to liking it here," I said. "I sure do."

Our strategy paid off, too, as we ended up the first half of the season, after playing all the schools in our league, undefeated.

John kept plugging away for the number eight spot and finally made it. And guess who won the deciding singles point in our closest match, against the only school that could have beat us?

None other than the absent-minded professor!

11

Long Beach

WHEN DR. EVANS ASKED ME IF I WOULD MIND COMING TO A meeting of doctors at the Research Institute, I said, no, I wouldn't mind, but brother, did I turn out to be wrong!

This meeting was called the Grand Rounds, and when I went down in the elevator with Dr. Evans and my mom to the lower level of the hospital, I didn't know what I was getting into. Dr. Evans opened a door and held it for us to walk in. Wow! This room looked like a Greek theatre! You wouldn't think there would be room for such a big place inside that building.

The circular rows of seats were occupied by men, mostly—there might have been a few women doctors there but to tell the truth I didn't notice. I wasn't looking at them; they were looking at me.

Dr. Evans gave me a straight chair to sit in facing them all. I turned all shades of pink. Then they started asking questions. They were told that I had just turned fifteen, and that this trouble had showed up when I was eleven.

"How much does he weigh?" somebody asked.

Mom was sitting in the front row, pretty close to me;

and that was some help. She told Dr. Evans, and he told them—142.

"When he was in the hospital three months ago he only weighed 100," Dr. Evans said. Then he told them what kind of pills I was taking, how much I ate, and so on.

"How is he doing in school?" somebody else asked.

Mom said, "Almost all A's!" Good old Mom, give her an opening to brag about her kids and she shoots off with all eight barrels. In fact, she can even do it without an opening.

"Is he as strong as ever?" was the next question. I decided to answer that myself. I didn't want them to get the idea I couldn't talk. "I'm a heck of a lot stronger," I said.

So far I had built up my weight-lifting, with the barbells I got for my birthday in February, to a record of forty-five righthanded and forty lefthanded.

But I still wanted to get out of there, and surprisingly enough, they let me. That was all there was to it.

I had a question I wanted to ask Dr. Evans, and I figured that was a good time for it, when he was thanking me for so graciously permitting myself to be stared at like a rare bird.

"Is it okay for me to play singles?" I asked. "In tournaments?"

"Well, I don't see why not," Dr. Evans said. "As long as you feel like it."

"Yay!" I yelled. "Come on, Mom, let's go."

She had to arrange for my next check-up, which involved some rather tight negotiation as I wanted to play in the Long Beach tournament the next two weekends. But Dr. Evans was still feeling grateful, so I got to go.

Going to tournaments is more fun than anything. You

either stay at motels with your parents, or you get "housing," which means you stay in people's houses in the different places where you go, and you ought to see some of those houses. They have swimming pools and tennis courts and thick wall-to-wall carpets even in the bathroom. One house we stayed in in Beverly Hills had thirty rooms, but I still haven't seen any homes I liked as well as ours.

You get to go to a lot of places like Disneyland and Pacific Ocean Park and Knott's Berry Farm that are fun; but Roy and I always stick to business and don't stay out too late any nights, as that can really wreck your tennis the next day. Roy is even more serious about that than I am—he made us walk out on a neat movie we went to one night in Santa Monica when I wanted to see it through to the end again.

Of course Roy, playing singles, and usually getting to the finals, would have to be more careful about that than I would, only playing doubles, which are usually played in the afternoon. But *this* time I was going to get to play singles too! Oh boy.

I broke the news to Dad as soon as we got home.

He broke right back with, "No—maybe next time— we'll see."

"But Dr. Evans said there isn't any reason I can't play singles now."

Mom stayed out of it, as she had promised she would when they made the Great Compromise. I wouldn't even have been able to play doubles in tournaments if it hadn't been for her.

But how strong do you have to get?

I was pretty disgusted with Dad for being such an old worrywart, especially when we drove up to Long Beach the first weekend for nothing, because it rained

Saturday afternoon; and all day Sunday I was as grumpy as a bear.

"If I'd been in the singles, I could have played!" I grumbled. Roy won his singles Saturday morning and didn't talk about anything else all the way home in their car. My parents were going to drive us up the second weekend. I could hardly wait—my school work didn't get done too well that week and I lost a match in chess. Laurie wanted me to play in another table tennis tournament with her during the Easter holidays and I said no, I was going to play tennis.

I was, but I could have been nicer about it.

On Friday I decided that I'd better just enjoy the doubles. We'd have a couple of extra matches to make up because of not having gotten them in the first weekend, on account of the rain.

I'd been wondering what I ought to give up for Lent, since Mom said it wouldn't be such a good idea to give up steak.

"Okay, I'll give up griping about the singles," I told Dad. "Just for Lent, that is."

We grinned at each other. My dad is a pretty good guy, even if he does worry too much.

And boy, what a weekend that was.

As soon as I got there, I found out that Jerry Cromwell who was number one in the Eighteen and Unders, was going to have to default in the doubles because his partner hadn't shown up. I didn't have the nerve to suggest taking his partner's place, but I sure wanted to. I was already playing in the Sixteen and Under doubles with Roy, but since I wasn't playing singles or mixed doubles I could easily take on another event.

I shot this agonizing look at Mom, who knew Jerry

pretty well because he is a friend of David's and has stayed at our house when playing San Diego tournaments.

Mom is pretty good at reading my mind, and she'll say anything she feels like to anybody, so she said, "Johnny could play with you, Jerry—he won the men's doubles in San Diego last fall with David."

"Hey, that's right," Jerry said. "How about it, Johnny?"

"Sure, I'd like to," I said.

So I played plenty of tennis that weekend.

Saturday Roy and I won two rounds in the Sixteens, and Jerry and I got a Bye, which means you move ahead without having to play, and then won the second round in the Eighteens. Sunday we would have both the semi-finals and finals of both events, if we made it.

My Dad said that was too much, I'd have to chose one or the other.

"It's only doubles," I said. "I could play doubles all day, and Dr. Evans said—uh—skip it."

I wasn't going to bring up the singles again, but I was pretty upset. I wouldn't have offered to play with Jerry if I was going to have to default. That would be terrible. I don't believe in defaulting.

Roy saved the day. He was a real friend.

"Why don't we just wait and see how it goes," he said. "Then if he has to I don't mind if we default in the Sixteens."

So Dad agreed that if the matches didn't turn out to be too tough, I could keep going.

Sunday morning there was a picture of me in the Long Beach paper playing doubles. I was up at the net, hitting a volley, but it was taken from the rear.

"That's all right," Mom said. "We don't have a whole lot of pictures of the *back* of Johnny!"

Roy and I just about cracked up, and even Dad had to relax that worried glare for a minute.

Luckily, Roy and I breezed through our semi-finals 6–0, 6–1 so Dad decided that was no sweat. But Jerry and I had to go three sets to get rid of our opponents in the Eighteens, and Dad began pacing up and down again.

Mom kept saying, "Wait and see—let's just wait and see . . ."

I felt great. Roy was the one who was half-dead. He won his singles, 16–14, 12–10, and after that he didn't have anything left for the doubles. Besides that, his elbow hurt so much he couldn't serve. I guess my dad could have made a point about singles, but he was kind enough not to. We lost the Sixteen and Under doubles in the finals, 6–2, 6–2; the only game we could win was my serve.

"I'm sorry, Johnny," Roy said, coming up with me to the net.

"Think nothing of it! Now Dad will let me play in the Eighteens." I shook his hand vigorously, forgetting all about his poor tennis elbow.

"Ouch!" he said.

"Oh gee—sorry about that."

We grinned at each other, and I shook hands with our opponents. Roy pointed to his right arm, and made a terrible face.

We all laughed.

Jerry had won the Eighteen singles with no trouble, and was anxious to finish up the doubles as he still had to play mixed doubles with Billie Jean.

We were playing the Tidball brothers; they are both

very good tennis players, and are the sons of a famous tennis player of the old days, who was watching us.

Jerry had been very nice to me all through the tournament. He didn't play it like mixed doubles, in which the man usually runs around taking all the balls he can get, even if he has to knock the poor girl over—he just played his half of the court and let me play mine. He even let me serve first in the easier matches, but he served first against the Tidballs.

Much to everybody's surprise, we won the first set, 6–1. I guess Jerry and I were surprised too, because the first thing we knew we were behind 1–4 in the second set, and the Tidballs were playing out of their minds.

However, we buckled down and after a terrific fight we won the set 6–4. Mr. Tidball said Jerry and I really put out a big fire.

Jerry said it was pretty rare for a fifteen-year-old to win the Eighteen doubles, and that he had enjoyed playing with me more than any other partner he ever had.

"You really use your head," he said.

Of course, I never could have won it unless I had Jerry for a partner. "It sure was nice of you to play with me," I said.

Boy was I happy! Roy felt great, too, after winning the Sixteen singles, and we whooped it up in the back seat almost all the way home.

It's over a hundred miles from Long Beach to San Diego, though, and it was dark, and we were sleepy. After that, we got to talking about more serious things.

Roy said he guessed he'd have to go into the Army in a couple years—or whatever branch of the Service he decided to choose if he didn't wait to be drafted. He could probably go to college, but he didn't know.

"It might be better to get it over with first," he said.

I thought about that—I hadn't thought much about it before. "I guess they won't take me," I said, "On account of this weird-o trouble I have with my blood."

"I guess not," Roy said.

I didn't want to fight. I wouldn't ever want to kill anybody. But I felt bad, too, because I didn't want to be different from the other guys.

I wished they would hurry up and finish that "new development" at Berkeley.

I wished it even more when I found a picture of Richard in the newspaper the next night. I called Mom into my room.

"That little boy we saw at the Clinic," I told her. "He died." I was awful sad.

She looked at me like she couldn't think of anything to say.

"You told me he was going to be okay," I said.

Mom took the paper, and sat down on my bed. I was sitting in my big chair, that they gave me for Christmas.

"That was what his mother told me," Mom said. "That's all I knew."

"Is that what I have?"

Mom closed the newspaper and began to cry. She cried so hard I was afraid she would break into pieces, and I went over and put my arms around her as tight as I could.

As soon as she could, she stopped crying, and smiled at me.

We both sat on the bed, and she told me that they really didn't know what I had.

"There are different kinds of diseases of the blood, and

all different kinds of medicines to control them," she said.

"I have to be able to trust you," I told her. "You have to tell me the truth."

She didn't say anything for a few minutes. Then she said, "Johnny, when you were eleven years old, Dr. Evans and his assistant told me that you could not possibly live for more than fifteen months."

Golly. I hope you don't ever know how it feels to have somebody tell you something like that. But it was kind of queer. The only thing I could think of right then was my parents.

"Gee, that must have been tough for you and Dad," I said.

"But they were *wrong!*" Mom said.

I thought about that.

Yeah—that's right. They *were* wrong. That was almost four years ago.

And I'd just finished winning the Eighteen doubles at Long Beach, when I was only fifteen.

"They sure were," I said.

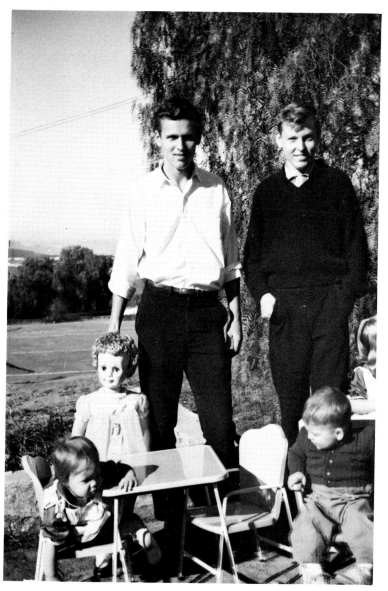

Rear: David and Johnny (age 14). Front: Teri and Bryan.

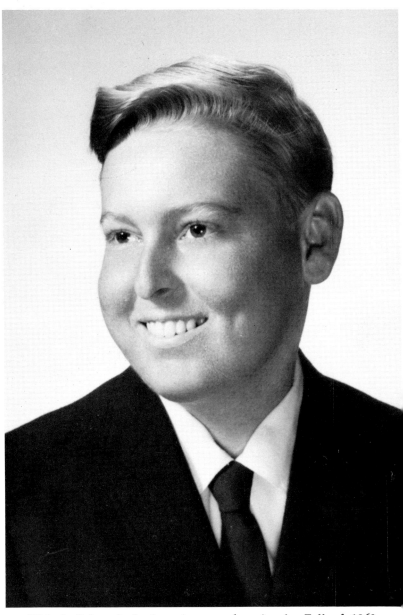

This is Johnny's Senior picture, taken in the Fall of 1962. Johnny was 15.

12

Questions

WELL, HERE WE GO AGAIN. I THOUGHT I WOULD AT LEAST be able to keep going until school was out.

This time was different from the other times when I had to have a transfusion. My red count was okay, but my white count began shooting all over the place and I had a temperature. It wasn't much of a fever and I don't know how my Mom even knew I had it but she stuck the old thermometer in my mouth and sure enough it was 100, so I had to go to the clinic even though it was the middle of the week.

Dr. Evans said they would like to keep me in the hospital a few days "for observation."

"Oh, *no,*" I said. "We have a varsity match the day after tomorrow."

"Well, which is more important? Your health or your tennis?" Dr. Evans sounded cross, and I felt pretty cross myself.

"It isn't *my* tennis," I said. "It's my team."

But I had to stay.

"It seems like the worse I feel, the madder he gets

at me," I told Mom. They had me all tied up in a hospital gown because I hadn't brought any pajamas along because I didn't know I was going to have to stay, and when you have one of those things on, you *have* to stay in bed.

Mom understood how I felt about Dr. Evans.

"He bawls me out, too," she said. "But I've noticed that he only gets cross when you get sick. It must mean he feels bad about it."

"Well, that's sure a funny way of showing his sympathy," I grumbled, but after that I didn't blame him anymore. It must be tough to be a hematologist.

"If you want," Mom said, "I could go buy you a pair of pajamas."

I sure did, and it was nice of her to think of it.

I really wasn't very sick, but the nurses kept coming in to take my temperature all the time. Since they will never tell you what it is, I acquired a great talent for reading a thermometer while it was in my mouth. This requires not only eagle eyesight, but flawless coordination of the teeth and good concentration. It never did go up to any more than 101, so I figured they would let me go home pretty soon.

We had a TV in the room and Dad and I listened to the ball games.

"When we go up to Berkeley," Dad said, "I'll take you to Candlestick Park to see the Giants."

That was the first I heard about going to Berkeley before school was out. I had been figuring on going in June, but that wasn't the way they were talking.

"Hey," I said. "What's the idea? I can't miss any *more* school . . . "

Mom said I didn't need to worry about my school work, I was two years ahead already and I could just forget about it until next year, and take it easy.

"*Forget* about it?" I said. "After all that work? No sir."

So that's why I went to see Mrs. Peterson before we left. She said she thought I was absolutely right, and she wouldn't want to see me waste all that work either. I had three A's and a B plus on my quarter grades, which was the closest I had come yet to my goal of all A's. The B plus was in English, and I was planning on bearing down on that during the last quarter.

"I can get the assignments from your teachers for the rest of the year, and you can work on them whenever you have a chance. You wouldn't have to finish them all by the end of school, even. You could have all summer," she said.

"Golly! That would be great. I sure would like that," I told her. "That's awfully nice of you, Mrs. Peterson."

"That's what I'm here for." She was trying to sound business-like but I could tell she felt bad that I had to go, because her eyes weren't twinkling the way they usually did.

"I'm sorry I have to let the team down," I said.

"You're not letting anybody down; you're doing a fine thing," she said. "And it's going to help a lot of people, just you think about that!"

Gee whiz, I thought, I'd better get out of there before she burst out crying.

When I got out in the hall I noticed that the bell had rung for first lunch, and as usual I gravitated toward Room 22. Everybody had their heads bent over their chessboards when I poked my head in, and I bet it was the quietest place on campus. Nobody noticed me for quite some time.

Well, I was pretty *near* the top of the ladder, I thought. A week before Easter vacation I had challenged Anderson for the number one spot, and we played all week. I was ahead of him by eight points, having taken a bishop, and I'd had hopes of finishing him off when I came back to school. It was sort of like David, I thought, at the Nationals. I *almost* made it.

Laurie would be the one who saw me first.

"Johnny!" she shrieked, so loud a bunch of guys jumped and somebody dropped one of their pieces.

Everybody looked up sort of foggily, and then smiled at me. Gee, they looked nice.

"Hey, Johnny, long time no see."

"Where've *you* been?"

"I didn't know you were coming today," Anderson said. "I already started this game with John——"

"Oh, that's okay," I said. "I didn't expect to play. I guess I won't be back in school for a while."

Laurie was standing next to me, and she put her hand on my arm but she didn't say anything, which is quite a switch for Laurie. Usually she talks all the time.

"Why don't you finish your game, Johnny?" John said, scraping his chair back.

"Sure, it's okay with me," Anderson said, and whipped out the little notebook we use to mark down our positions; before I could say anything he had switched the pieces on his board back to the game we were playing.

"Gee, thanks," I said.

That was sure nice of him. He didn't have to do that.

After only three moves, I made it. I was on top of

the ladder, and everybody was saying "Congratulations, Johnny!" and shaking my hand.

At first I thought it wouldn't be fair, because if I wasn't in school nobody could challenge me, but they all said it was fair, and I deserved to be number one. I had thought I would feel great when I finally got to the top, but all I could think of was what a great bunch of kids I knew. I sure was in a hurry to get that radiation deal over with and get back to school.

Laurie wanted to know where I was going, and I said up to Berkeley for some tests.

They would probably think I meant the College Boards or something. I hoped they would.

I wished that was what they were myself. I was getting scared.

Mom and Dad planned everything so it would be fun, driving up the coast. We were getting to stop the first night at Ojai so we could watch David playing in the Interscholastic Championships. All my friends in tennis would be there. And I didn't have a temperature any more. I was taking a lot of pills.

We had a big old Packard, which Mom and Dad took turns driving, and I had the whole back seat. I could go to sleep whenever I felt like it, which I did, some. I didn't exactly feel like playing tennis, I have to admit.

"I hope this operation or whatever it is will fix me up so I can play tennis whenever I want to," I said. I said that several times. And I asked about a million questions.

I don't know why I never asked questions before. I guess I was too busy playing tennis.

"Why do I have to go to Berkeley *now?*" I said. "How come Dad is getting out of teaching college? Why didn't we wait until summer?"

"We thought we might take you and Roy to the Nationals this summer," Dad said.

"You're kidding! Me and Roy?"

They almost had me sidetracked, but after a couple dozen questions about the Nationals, I switched back to Berkeley. It wasn't that I didn't believe them, because when my parents promise you something you can count on it. But first I had to be okay.

"Why can't I just go on taking pills?" I asked. "Why do I have to have this radiation? How are they going to do it? Will it hurt?"

Mom said the doctors up at Cal told her that it would not be painful. They did it by a new process of internal radiation, circulating it through you, which had just been invented by a young doctor from Mt. Sinai Hospital back East. He was going to fly out and spend his whole two weeks vacation just taking care of me. How about that?

"What about Dr. Vogel?" I asked. "Will she be there too?"

"Oh, yes, and Dr. Lewis and Dr. Mayne."

Dr. Lewis was in charge of everything; he looks like a grandfather, with gray hair, not much, and nice blue eyes. Dr. Mayne is tall and thin, with dark hair and brown eyes that crinkle when he smiles, and he has some children around my age.

They were the doctors that my parents went to when they wanted some hope, Mom said, and they never got cross. I guess they weren't afraid to get to liking me, like Dr. Evans was, because he kept thinking I was going to die. He had said that if my parents wanted to take me up to Berkeley they had better hurry up and do it. But they said there were a lot of unusual things about my case, and besides, you can't find a cure for anything if you don't try a lot of different things.

In case I am not being perfectly clear about all this, I can tell you I wasn't very clear about it myself. It was a big mystery. Nobody refused to answer my questions, but they sure didn't give out with much information. I decided I might as well wait and see what happened when I got there.

We had a wonderful time in Ojai, which is a beautiful valley north of Los Angeles full of huge prickly-leaved live oaks and orange groves, surrounded by high blue mountains, and in May there are flowers everywhere. In the middle of the valley is the little village of Ojai, which is the only town I ever heard of that is built around a park full of tennis courts—everybody in Ojai loves tennis.

High school and college teams from all over California were there—I could have been in it myself if I had been well enough to play. David and I both won some trophies there when we were younger, but David, as a Freshman in college, was not expected to win that year, except, naturally, by me and Mom, the incurable optimists. He played well and upset the top man from Berkeley in the second round, but after that he lost. We had a great time at the motel that night, though, playing cards.

The next morning David turned south to UCLA and we drove on toward San Francisco, taking the long way around, the Coast Route, because Mom had heard that nobody should miss the scenery. I said I would be in a hurry to get home, so we'd better see all the sights on the way up. Naturally I wasn't in a hurry to *get* there.

We drove along a winding road on a high bluff overlooking the Pacific. The colors of the ocean in Northern California seemed different—dark blue with patches of purple where fields of seaweed were floating just under the surface, and pale green in the shallow spots, with froth breaking over the jagged rocks. Some of the biggest ones were named—Morro rock and Jade Rock and one that was Spanish for White Rock. There were many headlands jutting out into the ocean, and the hills we drove along were covered with pine forests.

We got out of the car for a picnic lunch, and I breathed my lungs full of the fresh air and that sea smell mixed with the pine needles that Dad crushed in his hands for me to sniff. I collected a bunch of them for Frea to make pillows for Christmas presents—she likes to do things like that, and I'd like to have one myself.

At sunset, heading toward Half Moon Bay, I saw something strange—the sun, like a bright red nickel, rolling along the horizon with us as we drove northward, until finally it rolled out of sight behind the ocean.

The next day I would be in Berkeley, and I was getting scareder all the time.

13

The Box

DEAR ROY,

Just thought I'd write and let you in on all the gory details of my operation. For two weeks before the operation they were drawing blood and did two bone marrows (these aren't as bad as they sound, as they only take three or four minutes). Then on Monday the 14th I had a "trial run" which was supposed to help them to figure out how much radiation to give me on Thursday. First they stuck a needle in my right arm, then one in my left. Then they took me into this room where there was some sort of horrible machine looking me in the face. It was the box.

This "box" was about eight feet long, a little over three feet wide, and about five feet tall. It had glass sides and a narrow bed inside—for *me*. Underneath were two air conditioners; the box itself was pressurized, and there were all sorts of filters and radiation equipment on the end where my feet were, plus an intercom. In each window there were two big black gloves which the nurses used in taking care of me—as they could not get inside, of course, because of the radiation. There was a little sliding door they could put my food and other stuff in, then pick it up with the gloves and hand it to me. You probably have never heard of this before, mainly because it is the only one in the world.

The box, not quite made on the assembly line, costs as much as a good house! It has been used only twice before, so it is still an experimental thing. A doctor from New York who came to Berkeley *just* for my operation, invented the box. Anyway, I got in the box and they proceeded to "connect" me. Tubes coming from one end of the box were connected to the needles in my arms, while a blood pressure band was put on my arm. On both ankles and both wrists were elastic things like tight wrist watches and wires from them leading out of the box to an electrocardiograph. They also had to keep constant track of my temperature, and there being two ways of taking temperatures, they chose the worse way, and it proved very uncomfortable.

During the "trial run" I was in the box for six hours, and for the "real thing" the radiation was given for six hours but I had to stay in the box, still connected, for another fifteen hours. The doctors stayed all night, and I had Charlie Brown in there to keep me company and cheer me up—good old Charlie Brown! Everyone was surprised to see him there, and he never stopped smiling. I also got to listen to the Giants game.

During the first six hours my temperature rose to 104, yet this was expected. The operation destroyed most of my blood cells, although it could not destroy all of them without destroying me. However, by way of a thirty-minute transfusion, some of my mother's bone marrow was given to me. My dad offered to give me his, but they decided that hers matched better. It is hoped that her bone marrow will fight against my remaining bad cells. That was something that my bone marrow was unable to do. Then they did a skin graft, putting some of my mother's skin on my stomach to see if it would "take." If it does take, there is a better chance that this operation will fix me up for good

Since the radiation, they have been taking blood samples every day. I have to stay in the same room because, until my blood count builds up again, I could very easily get an infection. I am in "isolation." Everything in my room has to be sterilized, and no one can come in unless they scrub themselves clean, and wear special gowns and a mask over their mouths and noses (worn only once and then thrown away—so are the boots they have to wear). I have private nurses twenty-four hours a day while I am in isolation so the nursing and the room alone came to $1500, plus all that stuff they throw away!

My usual day goes like this: I have breakfast at 9:00 and a sponge bath at about 10:00. Somewhere in between they come and draw some blood. Then lunch is at 12:00 and dinner at 5:00. I have a TV and a radio, so I listen to the baseball games on the radio and also watch a lot of TV.

Have you got a doubles partner for the Southern Cal yet? They told us that we would be here until June 17th so our plans changed in a hurry when we found out I could go so soon. If you still don't have a partner you could put my name in, and it is possible that I could play. However, if you can get a partner, please do as it is doubtful that I could play, and I wouldn't want to leave you with no one. It is doubtful for two reasons—whether I'm really ready for it, and whether my dad will let me, and you know my dad! I might have a really great surprise for you, though, when I get home, so be ready.

I'm getting quite a few "get well" cards but the one I enjoyed most was the one from all the guys at Morley Field.

One thing I haven't done much of up here is homework. I wrote two compositions and a book report, and did some research on my term paper for English, and half of my Latin, but that's about all. By the way, how did you do on that Science test? Well, guess that's just about it.

Sincerely,
Johnny

I wrote this letter when it was all over, but I wasn't so cheerful to begin with, when I didn't know what was going to happen next. In fact, I was so grumpy all through the "trial run" that I never smiled once. Mom said it would be a lot easier on me if I wouldn't be so tense—but nobody told me how long it was going to last! After I was in there about a million years, one of the doctors told me in his jolly voice that it was "*half over*."

The bed I was lying on didn't fit me, so my back ached all the time—they had to massage it with those black gloves—and nobody mentioned until just before it was time that I was going to have a "little operation" at the end. This new doctor came in and cut out a small "node" in my neck in order to measure the amount of radiation I should have. Dr. Mayne told me this doctor was a great surgeon, and that it was like having a famous tree surgeon to cut off a little twig—but I wouldn't have cared, at the time, if he had been the President of the United States.

After that, the real thing wasn't so bad. Sol (everybody

called him that), the nice young doctor from New York who invented it, fixed the bed so it would just fit me; and I knew what was going to happen, so I took it in stride. An ordeal consists of one unpleasant thing after another when the patient doesn't know how long it will go on. The second time I knew exactly what was going to happen and that nothing would hurt too much: I just had to be patient. And besides, I had Charlie Brown in there with me. I could look at him and imitate that cheerful expression, so my parents would feel better. They were outside "the box," with a whole lot of doctors and nurses, looking at me all the time. Man, it was like in the zoo.

Afterwards, I was in the "isolation room" of the Donner Lab Hospital—they took the box out and left me in there. I was told that my morning, afternoon, and night nurses were all beautiful brunettes, but aside from the fact that they all had brown eyes, I wouldn't know. Nobody came into that room without wearing a starched green hospital coat and trousers, a green cap over all their hair, a mask over their nose and mouth, rubber gloves, and "booties." The masks, caps, gloves and booties were worn once and then thrown away in a special wastebasket in case they were contaminated by radiation. *I* was the radiation—each morning I got measured by a geiger-counter, and boy, did I tick!

I didn't have to wear all that stuff myself, thank goodness. I was pretty comfortable walking around, sitting in my chair, or lying in a superior type hospital bed that had electric controls I could work myself; it wasn't too high, hard or narrow. I had to wear a hospital gown, but I got resigned to it—I was so glad I didn't have to wear all that other stuff. My nurses and visitors had to wear it so they wouldn't infect me with anything because my resistance was supposed to be around zero, and everything had to be thrown away because even my perspiration was radioactive.

That's why I had to have all those sponge baths. I never had that many baths in my life—I hate baths. Showers after tennis, okay. Baths—only when my Mother made me. Now I was so white you couldn't tell which was me and which I was wearing.

My morning nurse was the tall one, with the biggest brown eyes. She was named Hilde, and my mom said she reminded her of a tigress defending its young. If there was a germ around, she'd get it before it got me. She made it clear that she did not approve of *any* visitors, but the doctors said it was okay for my parents to come in (properly sterilized) so of course my mom came in every day; after a couple of days my dad had to go back to college, although he said he would fly back any time I wanted him.

In the afternoon I had a short French nurse, and my night nurse was a regular baseball scoreboard, and very nice. A couple of times she finished my rosary for me when I fell asleep in the middle of it! They were all pretty young, and to be the nurses of a radioactive patient like me you had to be a special volunteer—because you were taking a chance.

Hilde had also been the nurse of the second boy they had in the Box, who was about my age. He had to stay in isolation 100 days, because he did get some infections, but he was doing fine now—back home again.

"It must have been awful hard for the first little boy that did it," I said to Hilde one morning.

"He was so young, they told him it was a ride in space." (She looked like a Martian, too!)

"They couldn't have told me that—I wouldn't have believed it," I said. "But it's nice to know that two other guys have been in there—and come out okay."

"Oh, they really take good care of you."

"They sure do."

A few days after the operation I had a bone marrow transfusion, which took only a half hour, and a skin graft, by the great "tree" surgeon. He took a piece of Mom's skin about the size of a postage stamp and brought it in to me—along with the skin came a message from Mom saying it didn't hurt much. Maybe it didn't hurt *her* much!

A few days later she came in to see me, and I said, "Thanks a lot for giving me your bone marrow, Mom, but I can't say I enjoyed that piece of skin. You sure are brave."

"I'm only brave about the things that don't hurt," Mom said. "Right now I hurt like the dickens, and I may burst out crying any minute."

She was holding her head stiff; she said she had an "LP headache."

"A long-playing headache?"

"That's a good name for it—actually, it's 'lumbar-puncture.' Some people get it when they have a spinal anesthetic; mmm—it hurts."

"Guess I'll have to reimburse you for that out of my blood money," I said.

"Blood money" was a fancy name for bribery. After the trial run, my parents said they would pay me $5 for each hour in the box, plus $1 for every "stick" I got, and varying amounts for other such gruesome details as suppositories, bone marrows, the skin graft, etc. That way, instead of thinking "Ouch!" I could think of my bank account.

So far my ACHE$ and PAIN$ included 28 needle sticks at $1 each and 26½ hours in the box at $5 per hour.

"I'm getting rich," I said. "You owe me $175 so far."

"Well, just don't hold out your grimy little fist for it right this minute," Mom said. I could tell from her eyes that she was teasing.

"Grimy!" I said. "You are looking at the *cleanest* boy in the *world.*"

"Don't make me laugh; you're hurting my neck!"

"Just look at these lily white hands," I said, holding them out. "Aaugh!"

"I wish I'd hurry up and feel like *me* again, instead of so miserable," Mom said when she left.

It made me feel better to have her complain a little bit. I got tired of everybody being so cheerful.

All the nurses would say, "Johnny is having the time of his life. He doesn't even have to comb his own hair."

Dr. Vogel understood. She was my special doctor, who came in every day. She never made jokes, and she was always so careful not to hurt me; once, when she couldn't help hurting, there were tears in her eyes, I think, although she wasn't the type of person who would cry.

One time when she was there the nurse went out, and she stayed with me. Even though I knew she had dark hair, her eyes were blue, and very quiet, like her voice.

"I'm glad you don't make any of those jokes about all the nurses taking care of me and me just lying here, being lazy," I said. "It isn't like that."

"I know."

"Could you answer some questions I've been thinking about?" I asked her.

"I'll try."

"Well—I've been wondering—why did I have to have all

that done to me? Why couldn't I just go on taking medicine?"

"Because the medicine stopped working, Johnny. That's what we found out when we looked at your bone marrow."

"You mean the "bad cells" Dr. Evans was talking about?"

"Yes."

"Well, if the medicine stopped working, why am I taking it again?" I sure was surprised to find those pills on my tray that morning. "Didn't the radiation get all the bad cells?"

"It got a lot of them. We're hoping your mother's bone marrow will take care of the rest. And the medicine will work again now."

"Oh." We didn't say anything for a long time. Then I *wasn't* cured yet.

I'd just have to go on fighting.

"Dr. Vogel," I said. "Is what I've got some kind of cancer of the blood?"

She wasn't supposed to tell me, I guess. "Would you mind if I asked Dr. Mayne or Dr. Lewis to explain it to you?" she said. The nurse was coming back in anyway.

She put her hand on my hair for a minute, and then went out of the room. I turned my head away.

It wasn't much of a surprise, I guess.

But I'm glad my parents didn't tell me when I was only eleven.

14

Isolation

MY DAD CAME UP TO VISIT US THAT WEEKEND. HE BROUGHT
back several book reports and compositions my English
teacher had corrected, and they were all A's.

I showed him a new one I had just written:

Essay on Ignorance

There seem to be two theories about ignorance. The
first is summed up in the saying, "What you don't know
won't hurt you"; or another way of putting it is, "Ignorance is bliss." The second theory states that ignorance
causes hatred, distrust, and fear. I feel that it would be
unwise to go along entirely with either theory. It depends
more on the persons involved and the situation.

In the first case, I shall consider an experience of my
own. When I was eleven, I was playing in a tennis tournament and lost decisively to a boy I normally would
have beaten. I felt very tired and we went to our family
doctor, who found that I had lost a lot of blood. Baffled
by the cause, however, he sent me to a blood specialist
in La Jolla. The specialist told my parents that I had

leukemia and could not live for more than fifteen months. We went to Berkeley and consulted another blood specialist who said that my condition differed in many ways, although he could not say exactly what was wrong. At the time, my parents told me none of this. I feel it is obvious, in this case, that it was better for me not to know. I was only eleven years old, and that knowledge could, understandably, have had a very serious effect on me.

The second example of ignorance is concerned with the Catholic Church. Among other things, some Protestants feel that Catholics are "idol worshippers." This is because, if they walk into a Catholic Church they will see a statue of Mary on the left and one of Jesus on the right. Since they probably know nothing of Catholicism, some think that Catholics must worship these statues and not God. The fact is, however, that these statues are to God as our flag is to our country. They are symbols, not sacred in themselves, but representing something sacred. In this case, through ignorance, non-Catholics would at least distrust the church, if not hate it. The point is, it is unfortunate that one should hate an entire religion because he does not know anything about it.

A third case of ignorance is that of white people who think that they are better than Negroes. Some, while "meaning no harm," automatically move away when a Negro moves in, refuse to serve Negroes at their restaurants, and refuse employment. Others, such as the Ku Klux Klan, actually threaten, beat up, and kill Negroes. Here is a type of ignorance that is very serious.

In coming to a conclusion about ignorance we must look at the persons involved. If a young child is ignorant, it may not matter because he has no responsibilities. He could not deprive a Negro of a job or refuse to serve one.

However, when he grows up, he will have to make these decisions. When this time comes, he cannot afford to be ignorant, for he has the power to hurt many people. President Kennedy, for instance, could not say with a clear conscience, "Well, I didn't know," if he was responsible for 100,000 deaths. Not many people have as much responsibility as Mr. Kennedy does, but practically every adult has a few very important responsibilities, and he cannot afford to be ignorant.

After he finished reading it, Dad said, "That's good, Johnny."

"There's something I want to know," I said. "I want to go to Heaven—but not *now*. But how do you know there is one? I mean, I *believe* it, but sometimes I wonder about it. And lots of people don't think there is. They think you're corny if you do."

"A great many intelligent people do think there is," he said. "As far as you can go back, men have believed in heaven. And it seems as if Christianity either has to be *all* true, or else it's the greatest hoax in history. You can't very well say that Jesus, who did exist—that is a historical fact—was a good man, but a liar."

"But what's it like in heaven?" I asked.

I knew what he'd say, of course. Nobody knows. I guess you have to go there to find out.

"Some great writers have tried to describe it," he said. "St. Francis de Sales wrote, "Represent to yourself a beautiful serene night, and consider how pleasant it is to behold the sky with all the multitude and variety of stars; then add to that beauty the glory of a bright day . . ."

I liked that. I wouldn't want to go where it is dark.

"I'll get you some books," Dad said.

But I kept wondering why, if it's so great in heaven, nobody ever wants to die?

I sure didn't.

I wanted to hurry up and get out of the hospital in time for me and Roy to go to the Nationals.

They said we could!

The doctors all said so. They said I had "great powers of recovery" and that playing tennis, and my *spirit,* was probably why I had been able to live all these years when nobody thought I could.

How about that?

Dr. Mayne explained to me that when you take the different kinds of drugs they are discovering all the time to fight these diseases, they work for a while and then your cells build up a resistance to them. He said I had some cells in me that were really tough. "We saw one of your cells that was different from any other cell any of us has ever seen," he told me.

"Is it really different from *any* other?" I asked.

"Absolutely."

"Ah," I said. "You'll have to name it after me."

I told him that I hoped what they had done to me would help to discover a cure, even if it didn't cure me. I would like to help little kids like Richard.

But Dr. Mayne said, "We've just been trying to save *your* life, Johnny. We've known you a long time and that's all we care about right now. We've been fighting hard— and you've fought the hardest of all."

"Gee, thanks," I said. Golly, they were all so nice to me. And they spent so much money. I kept trying to find out how much, but all I could extract was "In the thousands." They all laughed at me when I asked, but you can't blame me for wondering.

Everybody had always told us that I would be in there a long time, but all of a sudden, after only nineteen days, they opened up the door that had a big KEEP OUT sign on it and everybody started coming in and out with ordinary clothes on, and no masks. It wasn't June 17—it was only May 29!

My mother was still in the hospital, in the ward across the hall, because of her long-playing headache, and the first thing I knew, she was standing in the doorway in a pink bathrobe, with her hair showing, and she certainly did look pretty. I hadn't seen anybody's hair for a long time.

"Hey, Mom!" I said. "I'm *free!*"

Well, you will never believe this, but what do you think my mother did then? She began to cry. She came in my room and sat down in my radioactive chair, only I guess it wasn't anymore.

"I'm sorry," she said, "but I'm so surprised. Everybody's been taking such good care of us, and now all of a sudden it's all over. And Daddy isn't here, and I don't know what to do." Then she cried some more.

"Well, for Pete's sake," I said. "*I'll* take care of you. Come on, let's get out of here!"

They were letting me go stay with her in the apartment she had rented for a month, a few blocks from the university. My dad was in the middle of final exam week at his college, and I had to stay up there for some more tests at the clinic, but they said there was no reason for us to stay in the hospital.

Mom couldn't believe it. She kept saying, "But I

thought you had to stay there *much* longer—on account of infection." And she still had a stiff neck, so she couldn't drive the car very well, especially in "this traffic!" Dad had left the car there for us, and gone back by plane.

She said the cars all went so fast up there, so close together, that it scared her even when she could turn her head.

"Never mind. I'll be your navigator," I said, and I turned out to be pretty good at it—especially on parking, which it would have been impossible for her to do without me.

Finally I convinced her that I was really okay, and after that we had fun. We spent a large part of the day eating, as I was supposed to have six "small" meals instead of three, and I was so hungry that one day I had French toast for breakfast, a "snack" of an orange, doughnut, two milks and an ice cream cone, New York steak for dinner, a hot roast beef sandwich for supper, plus potatoes and gravy, more milk, desserts, etc. and then after we went to a great movie called *Murder She Said*, I had a hamburger and root beer! At that rate, I'd be up to 140 again in no time.

I was still horribly clean, but I seemed to have gotten used to it; Mom almost flipped when I told her she'd better buy me a wash rag. I guess that must have been kind of a shock to her. I also suggested a haircut—something I never did before either. But I wanted to look good when I got home.

We went shopping for some souvenirs and I sent word in no uncertain terms that I wanted a party as soon as I got home—with everybody there. I bought Mom a 99-cent straw hat to watch tennis in. We didn't either of us feel like playing yet but hoped to after we got home.

I guess I'm getting kind of repetitious ("after we got home") but that's all I could think about. In the ten cents store where I bought a lot of stuff for the kids, they were giving away goldfish, and Mom said, "Do you want one?"

"Well, sure—it's free, isn't it?" I said.

So we took it back to the apartment and put it in a glass pitcher on the coffee table, where Charlie Brown was sitting. He looked interested.

"Hey, that's just what Charlie Brown needed," I said. "A gold fish to watch."

"Well, this goldfish should be very flattered," Mom said, "because Charlie Brown is the best goldfish watcher I have ever seen. What are you going to name him?"

"I don't know yet," I said. "You can't decide a matter of such earthshattering importance in such a short time. We'll decide when we get home."

"You're going to take him home?" Mom asked.

"Well, of course," I said. "What else would I do with him?"

David was going to fly up from UCLA, after his last exam, and help Mom drive us home. "I'll be able to get my learner's permit in another month," I said. "Then I can help."

"I'll be glad when you do," Mom said. "I'll be happy to have you drive me any time."

"Thanks," I said. "I'm looking forward to it."

At my last check-up, the doctors at Donner Lab all said I was much improved, and wished me good luck in my tennis that summer.

Then after we got back to the apartment, and were packing our stuff, Mom asked if I wanted to send some candy or flowers to my nurses. I said yes, but there was one thing I especially wanted.

"I'd like to send some flowers to Dr. Vogel."

"To Dr. Vogel?" Mom sounded surprised.

"Get her some red roses," I said. "And Mom—there's something I have to tell you ..."

She looked up from the suitcase she was packing.

"I've been thinking about it," I told her. "And there are *two* things that I want. I want to get well—I want to go back home, and play tennis, and jump over the waves —but if I can't do that, I just want to go to heaven. Is that okay?"

Mom put her arms around me and held on tight and said, "Yes, Johnny. That's okay."

15

A Phone Call from San Francisco

I WAS STARTING TO PLAY TENNIS AGAIN AND IT SURE FELT good to be out on the court.

When you've played tennis as much as I have, it's hard to let two days in a row go by without playing, let alone four or five weeks.

It was great having Dave home. He worked on my ground strokes, showing me how to hit harder and closer to the lines, and he helped me straighten out my backhand. Arnell, of course, sat on the bench and watched. Mom said it wouldn't surprise her to see Arnell flying around the court attached to Dave's left hand while he played with his right. That's about the only time they ever let go.

But Arnell was a very nice girl. I wouldn't mind having her in the family. They said they were only "engaged to be engaged," but it looked like a foregone conclusion to me.

Roy and I were playing a lot of practice sets down at Morley Field, and I was finally beginning to click. One day we took on Dad and Carlos, who was the only boy my age who could beat me before I got sick. Carlos had curly black hair and had looked sort of bowlegged when he was little; his big brother said the reason he had such great reflexes was that he was double-jointed in his knees!

Roy started off like a house of fire, and I caught on after a game or so. At 2–1, for us, I followed my serve in, made a couple of put-away volleys, and won my serve at 40–0.

"Pretty good game," Roy said.

It was the first game I'd played like that since my operation, and I felt so good that we won the set 6–1. After that his parents came for Carlos, but we proceeded to demolish Dad and another good man player 6–0, with Roy playing lefthanded and me hitting a few of my patented behind-the-back shots.

"Looked like the mayor of old out there," Roy's dad said from behind the fence where he was watching.

Dad wouldn't let me play anymore, but I felt great. However, I was suspicious about one thing.

"What's the idea of not playing your hardest?" I challenged Dad. "That was pretty tough on Carlos!"

"You didn't think I played well?" Dad said, but the corners of his mouth were twitching.

"We could have beat you anyway," I said disgustedly.

Roy wanted to know if I could play in the Southern Cal doubles with him near the end of June. He hadn't asked anybody else.

"Wait and see," Dad said.

"*Wait!*" I said. "The deadline is Monday."

"Well, you're having a check-up Saturday."

"You don't have to remind me of *that*," I said. However, I was sure I was going to be okay.

"You said we could go to the Nationals, and if we're

going to the Nationals we ought to play in the Southern Cal," I pointed out.

"It would help us to get seeded," Roy said.

"Well, we'll see what Dr. Evans says on Saturday," was all we could get out of Dad.

On Friday at three o'clock I went to see Mrs. Peterson in the counsellor's office. I had not gone back for the last couple of weeks of school mainly because I could get my makeup work done faster at home; but I was going to take the tests.

"Well, Johnny!" Mrs. Peterson said. "It's good to have you back with us. You're looking fine."

"Thanks a lot," I said. "And thanks for taking care of my homework. I think I'm heading for that A in English unless I really foul up on the exam."

"I read some of your papers," she said. "They were good."

"Mr. Tanner has taught me a lot about writing," I said. "He figures out interesting assignments."

Mrs. Peterson was very anxious to have me attend the graduation exercises the next Friday as an "honor usher." The top students of the Junior class were to be ushers, and we were supposed to wear *tuxes*. Good grief.

"You can rent one at the Valley Valet Shop," she said.

I didn't think much of the idea, but Mrs. Peterson is about as easy to deflect from her purpose as an ocean wave, so I said okay.

"There's going to be a little dance afterwards," she said.

"Oh, no, you don't get me to any *dance*," I told her, and I guess she knew when she was licked.

Out in the corridor I ran into Laurie. To tell you the truth, I think she was just waiting there so I would, but she looked pretty good to me anyhow.

"Hi, Laurie," I said.

"Hi, Johnny."

She was wearing a green dress that looked nice with her hair. Anybody's hair looked good to me, after nineteen days in that space capsule, and I couldn't help remembering what David said about hers. "Wow, she's a blonde!" It was shiny and turned up at the bottom.

"You look thinner," Laurie said. "What did they do to you up there, anyway?"

"That's a long story," I told her. We were walking by the fountain, so I held down the faucet for her, and her hair dipped into the basin and got wet. She flung it back and laughed—she said it always did that, and it felt real cool.

"Are you going to be an honor usher?" she asked.

"Yep."

"So am I."

Laurie was a pretty smart girl in spite of the way she always acted. I guess a girl who was good in math and could play chess had to have *some* brains.

I told her my mom was waiting for me in the car so I had to go, and she said, "Well, see you at graduation!"

"See you," I said.

John was out by the old Packard talking to my mom. "I don't know what's wrong with you, but if it's not catching I'd like to come over and see you," he said.

"Hop in!" I said, and Mom said we'd love to have him.

As usual he had a paperback book sticking out of his hip pocket.

"Good grief, are there any books you haven't read?" I kidded.

"Well, what are pocket books for?" he said, not even cracking a smile. John had an unusual sense of humor.

He hardly ever got any of my corny jokes, but sometimes he would burst out laughing in the middle of a serious conversation. Then he would explain he had just remembered something he heard last week!

When we got to my house, my mom said perhaps he'd better call his mom and tell her where he was. He did, but he didn't get any answer.

I showed him the composition I wrote about my experiences in "The Box" so he would know that I wasn't "catching."

"Not any *more*," I said. "But boy, you should have heard me ticking after I first got out of there! You'd really think you had struck uranium."

He thought it was a good composition. "Lucid, and succinct," as he put it.

I happened to be watching my goldfish at the moment, and suddenly it struck me.

"Dart!" I said. "That's a good name for him."

"For whom?"

"For my goldfish. Naming a fish isn't the easiest thing to do, you know."

"I guess not," he said thoughtfully. "By the way, Johnny, I think you need a shave."

"A *shave?*" At first I thought he was kidding me, but then I put my hand up to my jaw, and sure enough, it did feel a little fuzzy.

How about that?

After that, I showed him my postcard ladder, which had just been turned upside down by an avalanche of cards from my grandmother and my mom's Aunt Bessie. First Aunt Bessie sent me 60, then Grandmother sent me 120, and then came another barrage from Aunt Bessie— 172—including quite a few from foreign countries. California was still in first place, of the United States, followed by Maine, Colorado, New Mexico, Michigan, Oregon, Arizona, Washington and Virginia as my Top Ten. I had some from every state, and North Dakota was in last place.

"You'd make a competition out of brushing your teeth," John said, shaking his head.

Mom poked her head in the door and reminded him to call his mom again, which he did.

After listening to the phone ring about fifteen times, he said, "Oh, that's right. My parents have gone to Los Angeles for the weekend. I'm supposed to stay with my Uncle George."

"Boy," I said, shaking *my* head. "How in the heck did *you* ever get to be an honor usher!"

We grinned at each other, and then my mom drove him to his uncle's.

"Next week I get my license!" I reminded her. In California, you could get a learner's permit when you were fifteen and a half—then you'd have six months' practice for the real thing. I could hardly wait.

What I *could* have waited for—indefinitely—was my check-up.

It was good to see my old friend Thelma, and I was delighted to hear that she had decided to follow my advice, and was taking up tennis.

"It's kind of fun," she said. "I didn't think I could do it at first, but I'm catching on."

When she started counting my cells, though, she almost fell off her chair. Apparently nobody had prepared her for the shock of seeing a real live person walking around with a white count of five hundred. From five to ten thousand is normal. Dr. Mayne had explained it to me—that the radiation had destroyed most of my good white cells along with the bad ones, and it would take a while to build them back up.

What surprised *me* was my red count. I thought she must have counted wrong. I felt *great*—but it was pretty far down.

Dr. Evans said I'd have to have a transfusion.

"Oh *no*," I said.

Mom was just as upset as I was, but she asked Dr. Evans if I could have it Monday instead of waiting until the end of the week, which he said would be soon enough. I certainly didn't want to have that hanging over my head, and Mom wanted me to be able to go to graduation.

"He isn't graduating, is he?" Dr. Evans said.

"No—he's a Junior, but they want him to be an——"

I shook my head at her, but she wasn't listening anyway.

"Whatever you say," he said, "I'm only the doctor around here."

I must not be in such good shape, if he was acting cross again.

"But I *feel* so good," I told Dad that night, after calling Roy to tell him he'd better get another partner for the Southern Cal.

"We can still play in the County Championships at the end of the month, though," I told Dad. "The Counties isn't like Southern Cal— we could win it easy. And I'm not even asking to play singles!"

"We'll see," Dad said. We were playing chess, and I started my horse off to capture his castle. I didn't feel like playing my usual slow, methodical game; I felt like *pouncing;* he might as well say no as "We'll see."

"What would you have done if *your* Dad would never let *you* do anything?" I asked him.

Dad anticipated my plan, and moved his castle. "I'm afraid my father was a worrier, too," he said. "So was my mother."

"Your father and mother *both?*" I said. "Boy, what a life you must have led!"

I took off after his other castle, and this time he was concentrating on a plan of his own, so after only twelve moves I plastered him. Boy, that was the shortest game I ever played with my dad. We started another, and Dad grabbed an early lead.

"How would you like to go up to LA and watch the Southern Cal?" Dad asked me. "We could stay at the Yucca Motel and have some fun in Hollywood."

"*Watch,*" I said. "Being at the tennis courts and not being able to play is like looking at a big juicy steak and not being able to eat it."

The phone rang, and Mom came in the living room to answer it. She looked surprised.

"It's for you, Johnny," she said. "It's a girl."

I figured it might be Laurie, but it wasn't. It was my morning nurse, Hilde.

She was calling Long Distance from San Francisco!

"Hi, Johnny," she said. "How are you feeling?"

"Great!" I said. "I'm playing tennis again."

"Well, I'm glad to hear that. I'm going back into isolation tomorrow. This time it's a little girl."

"Gee," I said.

"She's four years old—I'm *so* glad you're getting to play tennis."

My throat felt sore, and I got tears in my eyes. The poor kid.

"Tell her about *me,*" I said. "I really do feel great. I'm going to play in the County doubles with Roy—and I'm going to be an honor usher at Graduation next week."

"That's wonderful—I just wanted to know how you were."

"Tell everybody I'm okay," I said.

"I certainly will. And thanks for the flowers, Johnny."

"Oh sure. Thanks for taking care of me."

I tried to say goodbye, because I was worried about her money, but she wanted to talk to my mom, too. She didn't care about the money.

"That sure was nice of her to call me up," I said, after she and Mom finally stopped talking. I was glad Mom didn't tell her I had to have a transfusion.

My dad was standing by the piano, making a couple of chords with his fingers—not very loud.

"You can play in the Counties," he said.

"Oh boy!" I hugged the breath out of him.

"I may not be able to do much," I said. "But I'm going to do every single thing that I *can* do!"

16

The Counties

ON THE WAY HOME FROM THE HOSPITAL WE STOPPED AT the Department of Motor Vehicles where I took a test on the California road laws and got 100—it was a cinch, as I had studied the handbook all the time I was having my transfusion.

When I went up to the window, the man graded my test in about three seconds flat. He had me read the eye chart while he typed up the permit. I signed a couple of papers, put my voluntary thumb print on one of them, and he gave me my temporary license. It all happened so fast I couldn't believe it.

And then my dad let me drive the rest of the way home!

Boy, I sure was happy that day. When Dr. Evans came into my room to say I could go home, he had a big surprise for me—some new pills. This was a kind of medicine they never had before.

From what he said to my parents I figured it might work out like the first pills Dr. Evans gave me, which kept me well for over three years, and even if it didn't work that long, they were discovering new ones all the time. I could tell it was good news because Dr. Evans was so pleased. He was beaming.

"Well, Johnny," he said. "Off to the tennis wars?"

"Yes, *sir!*" I said.

On Friday morning they had a special assembly at Granite Hills; Mrs. Peterson called up to tell me I should be there.

It was the annual awards assembly, and it was held in the gymnasium, which is a multi-purpose gym: just like the tennis courts, they use it for everything else, because they don't have an auditorium yet.

The floor was so varnished you could just about see your face in it, and everybody was making a big noise banging the brown steel folding chairs, and about a thousand kids were all talking at once. I sat with John and Dick Kendale and the other guys on the team. They had a copy of the school newspaper which they were ripping to shreds.

"Hah!" Kendale snorted. "We finally got mentioned on the sports page."

" 'Our tennis team started out well,' " John read, " 'but had some disappointing late season losses.' "

"*Something* must have been missing," George said, grinning at me. I was sure sorry I couldn't have been there to help them.

"We'll win next year," I said. "And I think I'll take journalism and get on the staff—they don't know *anything* about sports!"

"Too bad Kendale has to graduate," Dennis said.

Kendale said he wished he could stick around a while longer. While I was gone he had worked up to the number one spot again, and all the guys liked him now. He won all his matches and they came in second in the League. Not bad!

When they started giving the awards, we all got our varsity letters—a big blue G. Kendale had been named on the All-star District team, and they made me an honary member of the All-Stars, besides being number one in the League in spite of not being able to play the second half. That was sure nice of them to do that.

It was a long assembly, because in a big high school like ours, there are so many awards, and it was a hot day. But near the end of it, I really woke up.

"For our tennis star and chess champion," Mrs. Peterson was saying over the loudspeaker, up on the platform, "a straight A student this semester and currently third-ranking scholastically in his class—I know you'll all be happy to hear that the Harvard Award for the most outstanding Junior boy goes to Johnny Sanderlin."

Gee.

Everybody was yelling, and pounding me on the back. I felt like crying but I had to get up and walk across the gym; my face was burning up. Mrs. Peterson shook my hand and said, "We're so proud of you, Johnny," and so did the principal of our school.

"Gee, thanks," I said.

I didn't know *what* to say, I was so happy.

That night my dad helped me get dressed in my tux. Boy, I would hate to wear one of those things every day. It had black trousers and a white jacket, a big black ribbon called a cummerbund which hooks around your middle, and a ridiculous little bow tie that sits on top of your Adam's apple!

But when I looked in the mirror I didn't look so bad. Now that I was taking the new kind of pills, I didn't have a fat face anymore, and I was almost as tall as David. Dave and I both wore our hair parted on the side, although his is darker than mine, and has a wave in it. Usually my hair is referred to as a "shock," but that night I combed it until it was really smooth.

My mom said I looked so handsome she wanted to take some pictures, so I let her, but I felt kind of embarrassed when I got to the gym. I got there early, so I could help seat the parents of the graduates.

Laurie was dressed up too, in a long pink dress, with white gloves up to her elbows, which must have been hot on a night like that, but she looked pretty.

She was on the other side of the gym, and didn't see me at first, but as soon as she did she started right over.

"Don't look now," John said, poking me in the side, "but guess who's coming?"

"Knock it off," I said. "Laurie's a nice girl. I like her."

I was surprised at myself for saying that, but I really meant it.

"Well, pardon me," John said in the high voice he uses for teasing. "I thought you didn't like *any* girls."

"Get lost," I said.

Laurie came up to me and said, "Oh, Johnny, you look so good in black and white."

"That's nothing," I cracked. "You ought to see me in color!"

She burst out laughing, and I felt great. It's kind of nice to look good for a change, and have everybody telling you so. After everyone was seated, we sat together in the basketball stands, and every once in a while Laurie would giggle. I think I've figured out why boys like girls who giggle. It's because they are laughing at *your* jokes!

"I have three Varsity letters now," I told her. "The

first year I was at El Cajon high school, so I got an E; last year and this year it's G for Granite Hills. What does that make me?"

"I don't know, what?"

"A good EGG!" I said.

The more she laughed, the more jokes I thought of. We really had a good time.

But then she wanted me to go to the dance afterwards.

"I don't know how to dance," I said.

"Well, if you can play tennis and pingpong, you can certainly *dance*," she said. "And if you don't know how, you ought to learn."

She had a point there, but I wanted to practice for the Counties and I was feeling a little tired, so I said I'd better not.

Roy met me at the Morley Field courts the next morning. I had my pajamas along because I was to spend the night with him. We had a lot of good practice, winning every set we played. Wilbur congratulated me on winning the Harvard Award, which he had read about in the morning paper, and said he was certainly glad to see me playing tennis again.

"What's the Harvard Award?" Roy asked when we were sitting around watching TV after supper.

I told him, and he was really impressed; that made me feel even better about it.

But then I remembered how disappointed Laurie looked when I wouldn't go to that dance. She turned her head away real quick, so her hair swung around and hid her face, but I could tell, and I really wouldn't have minded having her teach me how to dance.

But I was still afraid Dad would decide I wasn't strong enough yet to play in the Counties, and then we might not get to the Nationals. Not that he would go back on his word, unless I got sick.

But I wasn't going to get sick!

I'd be careful, and quit practicing if I got tired. I'd eat a lot, and get plenty of sleep.

I really took care of myself, and when Roy got back from the Southern Cal, where he was runner-up in the singles, we were all set to win the San Diego County Junior Doubles. We were the defending champions, as we had won the year before.

We breezed through the first couple of rounds, on the first and second day of the tournament, but in the semifinals, we struck a very determined team from La Jolla High, the Southern California Interscholastic champions. Ordinarily, this would only have made things more interesting, as, although Kripps and Johnson were a couple years older than we were, they hadn't been playing tennis as long as Roy and I, and hadn't had as much tournament experience. Kripps was a sun-bleached blonde surfer, and Johnson was a Negro whom I had played with quite a bit at the La Jolla courts; he was the most goodnatured tennis player I have ever run into, but *that* day he really meant business.

They won the toss, and elected to serve. Kripps won his serve easily and I told Roy to go ahead and serve first, since I wasn't up to my usual standards. He served well, and I put away a couple of shots at the net with no trouble—that was before I got worried.

But that was the only game we won that set. Johnson won his serve and then they broke mine. I couldn't seem to get my first serve in, and although I didn't make any double faults, I just didn't have it. They murdered my second serve.

I felt awful. Roy was tearing around the court, trying to win the match all by himself; he had to, I was *so* bad. How could I lose my serve?

"Never mind, Johnny," Roy kept saying, "We'll break back."

Instead of that, I netted a couple of easy volleys and lost Roy's serve for him, too. We lost the first set 6–1. I couldn't *believe* how bad I was.

Roy's dad was standing behind the fence watching. He took his pipe out of his mouth long enough to say "Come on, Tiger," to Roy, but he didn't say anything to me. I guess he didn't know what *to* say. I *never* played that bad before.

My dad was watching, too, but not anywhere where I could see him, thank goodness. He didn't have to worry about me going to the Nationals. *I* couldn't even win the Counties!

"Come on, Johnny," Roy said. "We'll take this one."

He was wrong. *We* didn't take the second set, *he* did.

The third set, I didn't feel quite so hopeless so I played a little better, but Roy played great. Kripps and Johnson also played out of their earlobes, and it was really two against one, but we hung in there, and at 9–8, our ad and match point in the third, I made my best shot of the day. It was also my most stupid. Kripps' drive was clearly going out, but I couldn't get my racket out of the way. However, I was lucky. By pure accident, the result was a perfect crosscourt angled forehand drop volley that hit the line.

"Yay, Johnny!" Roy pounded me on the back and pumped my hand up and down, but I never felt worse. It was all I could do to go up to the net and shake hands with our opponents.

Kripps didn't look too happy, but Johnson was grinning from ear to ear.

"Man, I thought we had you," he said.

"You played great," I told them. *That* was true enough.

Dad offered to let me drive part of the way home, but I didn't feel like it. I didn't feel like anything. Roy ought to go to the Nationals with somebody else. I was no good.

"The trouble is," Mom said, "You were thinking too much about how much better your partner was playing —that's always fatal. Sometimes it's one partner that's playing well, and sometimes it's the other. You may have to do the same thing for Roy sometime."

Mom always has these psychological theories about tennis which nobody pays any attention to, but maybe she was right. Anyhow, that's how it used to be, with me and Roy.

"If I could make a suggestion . . ." Dad said.

"Sure."

"You weren't on your toes. You don't have to *run,* just move your feet. You'll make a better shot if you do."

Can you imagine that? *My dad* telling me to *run!* Well, maybe not run, but step around. Be peppy.

Of course! I knew that. How stupid can you get?

And man, it really worked. The next day we won the finals 0 and 0.

"Hey, we thought we were going to beat you," our opponents said. "We're better than Kripps and Johnson, and they almost had you."

"Yep," I said happily. "*Almost.*"

All my friends were watching. Coach, my whole team, David and Arnell, Frank and Rol and my sisters, Roy's mom and dad, Wilbur, everybody. Even Mrs. Peterson came. And Laurie.

"Oh, Johnny!" she said. "You were wonderful."

Same old Laurie. I guess she wasn't mad at me after all.

David and Arnell were taking me to the movies that night, and David had said I could ask Roy or John to go along if I wanted to. Maybe I should ask Laurie.

If I could get up the nerve.

I asked David if he would ask her, but he wouldn't. He said I had to do it myself.

"You have to do it *sometime*," he said.

So I decided I would, and I did.

It wasn't so bad.

Laurie just said, "Sure, Johnny, I'd love to," and that's all there was to it.

They had some neat trophies for the Counties—about a foot and a half tall. They gave them out in front of the club house at Morley Field; with singles and doubles in all the different age divisions, both boys and girls, it took quite a while. The Tennis Patrons give great tournaments for the kids in San Diego.

Then Wilbur stepped up. He was all dressed up in street clothes, which I have never seen him in before, and he looked more like a plain business man than a hunter in Africa.

He was making some sort of a speech—about "achievement and determination under adverse conditions"—and somebody handed him this huge trophy which was big enough to hide behind.

Two minutes later, I was glad it was, because it turned out that it was for *me*. Everybody was clapping, and I wanted to sink through the grass.

"Golly," I said. "I don't deserve a trophy like that, just for being sick.

But Wilbur was shaking my hand, and beaming at me, and the more I thought about it, the better I felt.

I think that this trophy—I mean *I know* that this trophy

—will be a symbol of my fight to play tennis and win in spite of my blood condition; something more important to me than any tournament I ever won, even the time I played with David, and maybe even more important than winning the national doubles, because it represents a fight that has been going on for four years, and that will continue until I can win it.

I wished I could say something like that, but all I could say was, "Gee, thanks, Wilbur."

17

The Silver Ball

AT FIRST THE TRAIN WOUND THROUGH THE BROWN HILLS by the Pacific Ocean, the same way we always drove up to the tournaments in Los Angeles; but after eating dinner in the Union Station in L.A., we had to change to another train, and after that the scenery was different.

As we slipped out of the station in San Bernardino we climbed higher and higher into the mountains. Roy and I went up in the glass-domed car and sat at one of the little tables where you can play cards. We sat there until Nature turned out the lights, and we were in Arizona.

"This is a really neat trip," Roy said. It was the first time we had ever been anywhere in a train, and he was grinning all over the place—that special three-cornered grin of his.

Roy wasn't a very different-looking person—he had brown hair cut short in a flat-top crew-cut like all the other guys that year, and he was medium weight and medium height—but when he'd get to horsing around and teasing, he didn't look like anybody else but himself, his eyes twinkled so mischievously. Everybody liked Roy, because he was so full of fun, and nice to people. I was lucky to have him for a friend.

"I'm glad it's a good trip," I said, "because it's a long way to go for just one tennis tournament. What if we lose in the first round?"

"What do you mean, lose in the first round? We never lost in the first round in our life!"

He looked so indignant I had to laugh.

"Okay," I said. "We won't lose in the first round."

"We won't lose, period," he said. "But anyway, the Nationals is fun. You meet guys from all over the country—it's interesting."

"Just so I get to play tennis," I said. "I'd rather play and lose than not play at all."

"Sure about that?" Roy asked.

I thought it over. "Yep. I'm sure."

He thought about it too. "Well, I guess you're right. But if you *don't* win, you don't get to play the next round."

"Hey!" I said. "That's right. You remind me of that if I get too sloppy."

"Shucks," Roy said. "I don't see what you're worried about. If you can win the men's doubles and the Eighteen and Under, why worry about a bunch of kids?"

"You've got a point there," I said happily.

Gee, I sure was lucky, to be getting to go to the Nationals, and to have Roy for a partner.

We woke up the next morning in New Mexico, a beautiful green country where nobody lives for miles and miles. We went through the Raton tunnel, which is half a mile long and the highest point on the Santa Fe railroad, and then we were in Colorado. We seemed to be going on level ground, but a profile of the trip showed us that we were rapidly losing altitude, and it wasn't long before we could tell we were going down.

Once we got into Kansas, the scenery changed to flat land with farms spotting the countryside; and the square plots of land made it look like a king-sized checkerboard. Every once in a while we'd cross a river or go along the side of it for a while. Alongside of the Mississippi the tracks were scarcely higher than the river, and we went by the town where Mark Twain lived—Hannibal, Missouri. I bet he had a lot of fun when he was a boy.

Finally, we reached the outskirts of Chicago; it has so many outskirts and the train went so slow that I thought we'd never get into the station, but finally we did.

"Kalamazoo, here we come!" Roy said, and we grabbed up our suitcases and tennis rackets and ran—it sure felt good to stretch our legs after two and a half days of being cooped up on a train. Of course, we walked back and forth through the train a lot, but that sure isn't the same as being on a tennis court!

The national junior tennis championships for boys are played at Kalamazoo College; we stayed in the dormitory and ate at the cafeteria. It's a pretty place, with lots of green grass and trees, and the biggest tennis stadium I've ever seen, although of course Forest Hills is bigger. Guys with tennis rackets were swarming all over, and if you happened to overhear their conversation you never would hear them talking about anything but tennis.

Everybody from California was talking about the clay. Back in Maine where I played when I was seven years old, they had clay courts, but out in California all they had were cement, or some other type of hard-court, so I'd practically forgotten what it was like to play on dirt courts.

The kids from the South and the Midwest were used to clay, and everybody said they played a different game from the Californians. The main difference is that cement is fast and clay is slow—so the clay court players can get balls back that on a hard court you could figure on putting away. And another difference is that on a hard surface the ball always bounces the same way, but on dirt —especially after the dirt gets roughed up after several matches—the bounce can be really crazy.

"You sure have to keep your eye on the ball *here*," Roy told me. Of course he had tried it the year before. "But I don't mind it—it's kind of fun."

"Yeah," Carlos said, with a big grin. "You have to learn how to *slide*."

"I hear they're resurfacing these co'ts next year," a boy from the South was complaining. "As if we didn't have enough trouble with Califo'nia *now!*"

Roy and I went out that evening to practice, and Roy said I took to clay like a duck to water; it certainly is easier on your feet.

"You ought to try grass," a boy from Boston told us.

"I sure would like to," I said.

Wimbledon and Forest Hills are played on grass—the greatest tournaments in the world. But they are for men and women. Kalamazoo—the United States Nationals— was the greatest tournament in the world for Junior players, *and I was in it!*

Not only that, but Roy and I were *seeded*.

"Wow! Look at that," we said when we first looked at the draw. We turned to each other and solemnly shook hands.

There was this huge white cardboard sheet tacked up

on the bulletin board, covered with names of teams from just about every state in the Union, and up at the top, along with seven other teams, were our names in a special box. This meant that we were considered to be among the eight best teams in the country, out of a total of thirty-two. The other seeded teams were from Florida (two), Puerto Rico, California, Maryland, Georgia, and Michigan.

Of course, we might meet a team of "dark horses" in the first round, and be upset; that's the only trouble with being seeded. You are supposed to win, and if you don't, the team that beats you gets big headlines in the paper the next morning, and you just quietly slink away. Everybody says, "Hey, what happened to you? How could you lose to *them?*"

"If we hadn't been seeded, we'd have been dark horses," I told Roy.

"Yeah, and upset everybody in the tournament," he agreed.

We sure were happy. He was in the singles, of course, where he was seeded number four, and he won his first match without any trouble. Then we went out that afternoon and won our first-round doubles 6–0, 6–0. We attacked the net every chance we got, and both played great.

David was in the Junior singles (Eighteen and Under). He had been playing the preliminary tournaments, and there was just one boy he couldn't seem to beat—a boy from Arizona. Unfortunately, he kept bumping into him in the semi-finals, instead of being lucky enough to be in the other half of the draw, and that was the way it was in the Nationals.

"Well, you'll just have to beat him!" I said.

David grinned kind of worriedly. "Yeah—I'll try," he said.

The second day we won our doubles again, and the third day we had a little trouble—we lost the first set, but soon put out the fire and found ourselves in the semis. However, two bad things happened in the morning of that day. David and Roy lost their singles. If I could play singles I would be satisfied to be number three or four in the country, but of course they weren't. On second thought, if I were playing singles I probably wouldn't be, either—anyhow, not *right* after I lost. Roy and David are both good sports, but they weren't exactly happy that afternoon. David was still in the doubles, though, so he also had a doubles match to play.

His match was on the court next to ours, which wasn't going to help my concentration, although of course I would *try* not to listen to his score. But I sure was hoping he'd win the doubles so he would feel better.

We were playing a team from Florida which consisted of the boy who was in the singles finals—not the one who beat Roy but the other semifinalist winner—whose name was Bill, and a partner who wasn't quite as good as he was, but who was no pushover. His name was Ed.

Bill was full of beans, as he had just won a big victory, whereas Roy—who had given it everything he had and lost 8–6 in the third—was tired and disappointed. Of course, Roy and I have been in this same position before, and if you don't win the singles you're all the more anxious to make up for it by winning your doubles, so I figured he'd be okay.

Personally, I never felt more like playing tennis in my life. Roy told me to serve first, so I did, and won my

serve. My overhead was going great. Bill then won his
serve, and it was Roy's turn. He sure tried—the score
went to deuce about twenty times—but in the end we lost
the game.

"I can't serve," Roy said. "I can't hit *anything.*"

"Remember me at the Counties," I reminded him, and
he gave me a sickly grin. We almost broke Ed's serve,
but every time we got an ad, Roy missed his shot, and
every time he missed it, the more hopeless he got. In
his frame of mind, it would have been better if I had
been playing the ad court, but I always play the forehand side, and this was no time to change.

We lost the first set 6–4, and I couldn't help hearing
the umpire over in David's court announcing that he had
lost his first set, too. In the boys' division, we play two
out of three sets, but the older guys go three out of five,
in the semis. I managed to bump into Dave at the net
post while we were changing courts and told him to get
in there and *win!*

He was walking around like a bull with his head down
and a scowl on his face, but when I said that he looked
up and grinned.

"Okay," he said. "That's a good idea."

When you are tired, it's hard to concentrate, and I
noticed as we began the second set that Roy was letting
his eyes wander over to David's match every once in a
while.

"Come on, Tiger," I said. "Let's win this point."

In tennis, the best way to concentrate is to forget the
score, forget the way you are playing, forget everything
in the world except that you have to win *this* point. Then
if you don't, forget it and win the *next* one.

Roy knew that just as well as I did, but he didn't seem

to have it that day. The harder he tried—because he sure was *trying*—the worse he played, and we got behind 5–2, match point, in the second set. Roy was serving and it was ad out. Bill returned the serve with a vicious drive straight at my chest, but I managed to get my racket on it and dumped the ball back over the net. Bill was so surprised he just stood there, and it was deuce again.

The next point Ed got over my head in a perfect lob, and Roy raced over to get it, but hit it into the net, so it was their ad again. This time Bill decided to keep the ball away from me, so he hit it crosscourt, but I poached, and angled it off into the alley. I was fighting for our lives, and Roy appreciated it, but in trying to give me some help he was too anxious, and overhit.

I don't know how many match points we saved—somebody said afterwards it was eleven—but all of a sudden I got sick to my stomach. I went over to the fence and let go. Then I went back on the court.

That isn't the first time that has ever happened to me, so it didn't bother me much, but it did shake up our opponents. However, steady Eddie dumped Roy's serve back, it just rolled over the net and they had the ad again. I was still a bit shaky, but just then The Tiger came to life. Bill lobbed the ball over my head but Roy charged over to the corner and made a running cross-court forehand drive that split the baseline at Ed's feet. Ed scooped it up in a miraculous get and lobbed again. It was a weak lob, which was going to bounce right in the middle of the court, so Roy decided to take no chances on hitting it in the air. If he let it bounce first, he could kill it—but he forgot about that clay. The middle of the court was all plowed up by that time, and the ball gave a dull thud. "I guess that's it," I thought, game, set, and match for the team from Florida."

But the Tiger was not giving up. The ball bounced up about a foot and he got his racket under it and stabbed it over—wow! We won the next two points while they were still gasping. So it was 5–3.

We still had one big hurdle to get over—we had to take Bill's serve and it was the best in the nation in the boys' division.

But we took it, and after that—with Roy still booming away with those hard drives, and me putting away everything they hit up in the air—we didn't have much trouble winning my serve, Ed's and Roy's again to take the second set 7–5.

The third set was no cinch, however, and I was a little tired. I didn't play badly and I didn't complain about it, but Roy could tell, and it seemed to be just what he needed. I never saw him play better; we won the third set and the match—4–6, 7–5, 6–4. We were in the Finals!

"Thanks to you," Roy said. That's when they told us about those eleven match points—I guess I did save most of them, but another day it would have been Roy. And he had dug that impossible shot out of the dirt.

"We're a good team," I said.

"You can say that again!" Roy tossed his racket in the air and caught it. "And we're going to win tomorrow!"

David lost his doubles. I felt bad about that, but I was trying to cheer him up. We were sitting in the empty stadium, the sun was going down, and they were lowering the flag.

"You're a lot better than I am," I said. "I just got lucky."

"You could call it luck," Dave said. "But there are different kinds of luck. It's lucky if you have the skill and the brains and the opportunity to be a champion—it's what you do with them that counts."

"Well, you sure had bad luck last year," I said.

"I still could have won *this* year."

"So okay—you can win next year. You can win the singles at Wimbledon!"

"I'm sorry, Johnny," he said. "I'm spoiling all your fun."

"No, you're not," I said. "Because I don't think it's the most important thing in the world just to win a game. I used to, but I don't anymore."

I thought about how upset I was when Mr. Gordon took away my chess pass so I couldn't get to the top of the ladder. That seemed like a long time ago.

"You sure have grown up a lot lately," Dave told me.

"Hey, I don't want to grow up *too* fast," I said. "I still want to win that silver ball!"

"Well, whatever you do," Dave said, "you're a real champion."

I thought about that the next day when we walked out on the red clay courts to play our finals. It was a cool, clear day with the flag whipping in the breeze, and the stadium was filled with people from all over the country. We were playing two boys from Georgia who had upset the second-seeded team by lobbing every ball over their heads until they cracked up.

Roy and I had the advantage of being prepared for those tactics, so we had practiced our smashes all morning; but we were pretty nervous when we found ourselves in the finals. My overhead is supposed to be my best shot, and Roy makes such hard drives that all our opponents can do, usually, is to pop them up in the air, and then I put them away. With a couple thousand people watching, though, I broke out in a cold sweat. "Suppose I miss it?" I thought, when I saw that first moon shot go arching up into the sky. After all, they did upset their opponents yesterday. I reached my arm way up, the way David taught me, and kept my eye on the ball. "Crash!" I brought it down, and smashed the ball to the baseline. They lobbed it back up, and I smashed it again —this time they didn't have a chance. And Roy did the same thing. Sometimes we angled them into the alley, sometimes we smashed them deep to the baseline—in the middle, where the poor guys cracked their rackets together, both trying to return the ball at once; and on match point I made a perfect stop-volley that just dropped over the net and died.

Boy, that sure was fun!

We won the match 6–0, 6–1, and everybody cheered. Roy was hugging me and pounding me on the back, and saying, "Hey, Johnny, we're number one in the United States!"

I turned pink, as usual, and couldn't think of anything to say. I always turn pink when I'm happy.

Then they gave us each our silver ball.

It isn't even as big as a marble, but nobody gets it unless he wins a U.S. championship in Tennis.

"Boy, I sure am lucky," I said. "I wouldn't want to be anybody else in the world but me."

18

The Last Chapter

THIS STORY REALLY HAPPENED. IT WAS TAKEN FROM THE *diary and weekly newspaper of Johnny Sanderlin, who won the National Boys Doubles Championship with Roy Barth, two years after the doctors told his parents that he could not possibly live for more than fifteen months. A few changes have been made, chiefly in the order of the events, so that the book could be more unified, as told by Johnny himself the year he was fourteen.*

Actually, he and Roy won the Boys Thirteen and Under Doubles in 1960, the first year that U.S. championship was held, in Chattanooga, Tennessee, although they also played in the Boys Doubles at Kalamazoo in the fifteen year old division. The following year, the divisions were changed to Twelve, Fourteen, and Sixteen and under, and that is what they have been since. In the book, they are referred to that way in order to prevent confusion.

Johnny himself wrote the account of his experiences in "The Box" and he really said—after it was over and he knew he was not cured—"I wouldn't want to be anybody else in the world but me."

And it was not at Berkeley, but in another hospital, a few days before his sixteenth birthday, that he asked, "What's it like in Heaven?" After a philosophical discussion with a priest in a blue bathrobe, who came in from another room, he smiled and said, "Not that I think I'm in any immediate danger of death. I'm more optimistic than that!"

He had been very ill for two weeks—too weak to eat or drink and unable to sleep because of a pain in his chest. But some of his friends came in to visit him with their tennis rackets from the courts across the street, and he managed to get into a wheelchair so that he could go down to the end of the corridor and look out the big windows at the ocean every evening. He watched it until after it was dark and he could barely see the white froth of the breakers coming in. That may have been why he said, when asking about what happens after you die, "I don't want to go where it is dark."

He was notified that he had won a scholarship to college that week, on the basis of the Scholastic Aptitude Test he had taken December 3, so it was a very intelligent fifteen year old who said to his parents, "There are two things I want. I want to live . . . but if I can't do that, I just want to go to heaven."

Early the next morning, Johnny died.

He had lived every minute of his life—doing "everything he could do." And he was always a good sport, even when it came to dying.

I wrote this book because I thought it might help people. A girl in Canada who read an article I wrote about Johnny sent me a letter. She had been in an accident and crushed her foot. She said she hadn't been able to walk; she felt so bad she wouldn't even try. When she

read about how hard Johnny had fought, she was a-
shamed of herself; and now she told me she could not
only walk; she was "even dancing!"

Johnny would like that.

I can't think of any better way to end this book than
with the memorial page in his high school Annual.

From *Pageant*, Granite Hills High School Yearbook, 1963.

JOHNNY

When Johnny Sanderlin died this year after a long
battle with leukemia, we lost one of the finest boys ever
to attend Granite Hills. A modest boy, his quiet smile
and shock of sandy-colored hair made him a popular and
well-known figure on campus. A National Doubles Cham-
pion in tennis, he filled his home with trophies marking
his rise as a tennis star. He never raised his voice in anger
and was at all times willing to help others. . . . A senior,
Johnny maintained an "A" average scholastically and
qualified for numerous scholarships. Most of his classmates
never knew he had leukemia, and his fortitude will forever
stand as a monument to heroism.